- doctor yourself
- 1930's - Columbia Univ - cured polio
- High dose Vit C

VITAMIN C:
The Real Story

The Remarkable and Controversial Story of Vitamin C

Steve Hickey, PhD,
and Andrew W. Saul, PhD

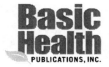

Basic Health
PUBLICATIONS, INC.

The information contained in this book is based upon the research and personal and professional experiences of the authors. It is not intended as a substitute for consulting with your physician or other healthcare provider. Any attempt to diagnose and treat an illness should be done under the direction of a healthcare professional.

The publisher does not advocate the use of any particular healthcare protocol but believes the information in this book should be available to the public. The publisher and authors are not responsible for any adverse effects or consequences resulting from the use of the suggestions, preparations, or procedures discussed in this book. Should the reader have any questions concerning the appropriateness of any procedures or preparation mentioned, the authors and the publisher strongly suggest consulting a professional healthcare advisor.

Basic Health Publications, Inc.
www.basichealthpub.com

Library of Congress Cataloging-in-Publication Data

Hickey, Steve

    Vitamin C : the real story / Steve Hickey and Andrew W. Saul.
      p. cm.
    Includes bibliographical references and index.
    ISBN 978-1-59120-223-3 (Paperback)
    ISBN 978-1-68162-888-2 (Hardcover)

  1. Vitamin C—Therapeutic use. 2. Orthomolecular therapy.
3. Vitamin therapy. I. Saul, Andrew W. II. Title.

  RM666.A79H53 2008
  615'.328—dc22

                  2008028974

Editor: John Anderson
Typesetting/Book design: Gary A. Rosenberg
Cover design: Mike Stromberg

Contents

In memory of Dr. Robert F. Cathcart III,
one of the most innovative physicians
in orthomolecular medicine.

Acknowledgments

We would like to thank Dr. Abram Hoffer, M.D., Ph.D., for his continued encouragement and support. Dr. Hoffer has played a leading role in ortho-molecular medicine, and he is an inspiration for scientists and physicians interested in nutrition and medicine. The late Dr. Robert F. Cathcart III has similarly been at the forefront of the use of vitamin C in orthomolec-ular medicine and has provided essential information used in compiling this book. Drs. Ron Hunninghake, Michael Gonzalez, and Jorge Miran-da-Massari of the RECNAC initiative have generously given of their time in keeping us informed of clinical work in vitamin C and disease. In the United Kingdom, Dr. Damien Downing has given access to his wealth of experience in nutritional medicine. Dr. Gert Schuitemaker, president of the International Society for Orthomolecular Medicine, kindly provided video and literature on Linus Pauling and his role in the vitamin C controversy. Drs. Hilary Roberts and Len Noriega have consistently given their scien-tific expertise to facilitate our understanding of vitamin C and its actions.

Any book on vitamin C and orthomolecular medicine owes a debt of gratitude to those individuals who endeavor to maintain the public pro-file of the background research. These include medical journalist Bill Sardi, Owen Fonorow of the Vitamin C Foundation, Rusty Hodge of the C for Yourself website, and Chris Gupta. We owe thanks to many more people, far too many to list here, for their efforts in preventing the vitamin C story from being completely hidden from the public.

Foreword

About forty years ago, I met Drs. Linus Pauling and Irwin Stone at a meeting in New York City. Linus Pauling spoke about his discovery of the structure of the hemoglobin molecule. During his presentation, he remarked that he wished he would live another twenty-five years because the future of new findings would be so interesting. Little did he realize that this wish and our meeting would change his life and give him thirty years. Dr. Stone told me about his interest in vitamin C, which he preferred to call ascorbic acid. It had saved him after a life-threatening motor vehicle accident. He had a massive collection of vitamin C reprints and I urged him to write a book.

After he got home, he wrote to Dr. Pauling and advised him that if he too took this vitamin, he would get his twenty-five years. This interested Dr. Pauling and he followed Dr. Stone's advice. To his surprise, his frequent colds vanished. Eventually, he was taking 18 grams daily. He used that number, which was 200 times the Recommended Dietary Allowance (RDA), and loved to tell everyone about it. Dr. Stone eventually published his wonderful book *The Healing Factor*.

Critics often are unaware of unintended consequences. At another meeting, Dr. Pauling suggested that ascorbic acid might decrease the ravages of the common cold. Dr. Victor Herbert, spokesperson for the anti-vitamin establishment, demanded evidence. Dr. Pauling thought that was fair and did a complete literature search. He found plenty of evidence, but Dr. Herbert refused to look at it. Linus Pauling's book *Vitamin C and the Common Cold* was a best-seller, and sales of vitamin C skyrocketed.

I was fascinated. Ascorbic acid was already part of the nutritional treatment program I used for schizophrenic patients, in combination with vitamin B_3. Starting in 1952, I used vitamin C as an antioxidant to decrease the oxidation of adrenaline into psychosis-causing adrenochrome. Schizophrenia is one of the severest of oxidative stress conditions. I also found that some of my schizophrenic patients who also had cancer began to respond to the large doses of vitamin C. Sarcomas are particularly sensitive to large doses of vitamin C.

I subsequently met Dr. Robert F. Cathcart III and studied his findings that high doses of oral ascorbic acid, as close to the laxative level as possible, were effective for treating cancer. He was also giving patients huge intravenous doses for a large variety of conditions. One of my patients with cancer increased her vitamin C dose as high as she could and eventually was taking 40,000 milligrams each day. Six months later, her tumor was no longer visible on a computerized tomography (CT) scan, and she lived another twenty years. This recovered patient changed my professional life away from a purely psychiatric practice. Physicians began to refer their terminal patients to me in droves, and since then I have seen about 1,500 patients. The results of my treatment have been generally good, much better than the results of surgery, radiation, and chemotherapy used alone or in combination.

The results of high-dose intravenous ascorbic acid are even more impressive. Dr. Hugh D. Riordan had more experience treating cancer patients in this way than any other physician. He showed that very high doses of vitamin C were something oncologists had only dreamed of: a chemotherapy that killed only cancer cells and left normal cells alone. He is honored by the new Chair created by the University of Kansas, where Jeanne A. Drisko, M.D., is Riordan Professor of Orthomolecular Medicine and Research. She is investigating the safety and efficacy of antioxidants, including vitamin C, in newly diagnosed ovarian cancer.

Considering the properties of vitamin C in the body, it is not surprising that it has proven so valuable. I will list only three very important roles, as you will read about the rest of them in this book:

- Antioxidant—Without antioxidants, we would slowly burn up from the oxygen in our atmosphere. It is essential that the body keep oxidation under control.

- Collagen formation—Collagen is an important structural protein in the body's connective tissues. Lack of vitamin C is why, in scurvy, the collagen tissues break down so severely.

• Histamine scavenger—Each molecule of vitamin C destroys one molecule of histamine. The bleeding tissues and loosening of collagen fibers
in scurvy is caused by the massive buildup of histamine in the body,
which does not contain enough vitamin C.

Vitamin C is very safe. It has always puzzled me why the medical profession was so eager to invent so many toxic properties when vitamin C
does not have any. False factoids are prevalent, and the profession still
considers these myths to be truth—something that could change with an
examination of this book. For example, vitamin C does not cause kidney
stones or pernicious anemia, and it does not make women sterile. Vitamin
C did not shorten Linus Pauling's life, as Victor Herbert claimed. Dr. Pauling lived eighteen years longer taking vitamin C than Dr. Herbert did without it.

Dr. Stone stated over and over that vitamin C should be classified as an
important nutrient that we need in quantity and cannot make, and not as
a vitamin. If you want to be really healthy, you should take enough vitamin C. After reading this book, you will know why and how much. I am
ninety years old and I have been taking vitamin C for over fifty years, and
I plan to stay on it forevermore. It has also been very good for my patients
but not so good for my practice—my patients get well too fast.

—Abram Hoffer, M.D., Ph.D.

Preface

Research into vitamin C is progressing rapidly, despite a lack of funding from conventional medicine for studies into its clinical applications. As you will see, vitamin C (ascorbic acid) has proven highly successful as an antioxidant for infections, the common cold, heart disease, and cancer. And even in very high doses, vitamin C is safe and nontoxic, in spite of any scare stories you may have heard in the media.

The purpose of this book is to tell the story of how the controversy about vitamin C has grown and continues while the increasing evidence demonstrates the value of the orthomolecular (megavitamin) approach. The story looks at the courageous efforts of pioneering scientists and physicians in vitamin C research. It also involves an understanding of political and economic influences in modern medicine. And finally, there are the astounding results of vitamin C studies, which demonstrate the effectiveness of this remarkable molecule.

Since its origins several decades ago, orthomolecular medicine, which uses nutrition to protect against or cure disease, has been regarded as highly controversial by the medical establishment. This rejection of the orthomolecular approach has little basis in science and reflects a bias at the heart of the status quo. In this book, we illustrate how the claims for vitamin C have been a central area of contention between conventional and orthomolecular medicine.

The disparity between encouraging clinical reports on vitamin C and paltry follow-up research is enormous. Well-documented clinical results indicate that massive amounts of vitamin C are an effective antibiotic against both viral and bacterial infections, a nontoxic anticancer agent that puts conventional chemotherapy to shame, and also a cure for heart disease. These claims are considered absurd by conventional medicine, a view that is totally without scientific support. By not performing or funding essential experiments on the clinical role of orthomolecular levels of nutrients, the establishment continues to avoid scientific reality.

It is our contention that, someday, medicine without vitamin C therapy will be compared to childbirth without sanitation or surgery without anesthetic.

CHAPTER 1

A Remarkable Molecule

*"Insanity: Doing the same thing over and over again
and expecting different results."*
—ALBERT EINSTEIN (ATTRIBUTED)

Vitamins are essential, because without them people will suffer ill health
or even death. Since vitamins are defined as being indispensable, they
are all, in a sense, equally important. However, some are needed in larger, more frequent amounts than others. Our experience of asking nutritionists which single nutrient they would take, if limited to just one, was that
nearly all picked vitamin C. This is not just a result of the popularity of
this vitamin, but reflects its widespread role in health and disease.

A full account of vitamin C takes us on a tour of evolution as well as
recent human history and takes in psychology and the social control of
institutions. Vitamin C provides a window into the errors and misconceptions that abound in conventional medicine. The real story of vitamin C
lies not only in the story of courageous physicians and scientists willing
to bring out the truth, but in the pressures and mechanisms on doctors that
make following a scientific path so difficult.

Vitamin C Basics

Vitamin C is a small molecule, a white crystalline substance similar in
structure to glucose. It consists of a single molecule, called ascorbic acid
or ascorbate, composed of six carbon atoms, six oxygen atoms, and eight
hydrogen atoms, all linked together by chemical bonds. It is a weak acid
and has a slightly sour taste, but many food supplements use salt forms
(sodium ascorbate, calcium ascorbate, or magnesium ascorbate), which

1

are neutral or slightly alkaline rather than acid and can be easier on sensitive stomachs. Ascorbic acid is about as acidic as citrus fruit or a cola soft drink. Some vitamin C is in our food (especially fruits and vegetables), but a normal diet does *not* provide sufficient quantities for optimal health.

Vitamin C has many functions within the body. Bone and its connecting ligaments and tendons receive their strength from a long, stringlike protein molecule called collagen. Collagen is a structural protein, which acts like the embedded fibers in fiberglass composites. Vitamin C is vital to the body's production of collagen. Absence of vitamin C causes scurvy, leading to spongy gums, loosened teeth, bruising, and bleeding into the mucous membranes. Several of these symptoms are caused by loss of collagen and connective tissue from blood vessels, which then become fragile and unable to respond to blood pressure and other stresses.

Vitamin C plays a role in protecting the brain and nervous system from detrimental effects of stress. Synthesis and maintenance of the chemical messengers (neurotransmitters) adrenaline (epinephrine) and noradrenaline (norepinephrine) depends on an adequate supply of vitamin C. These neurotransmitters are vital to brain functioning and affect people's mood. They function as stress-signaling hormones and are produced in the adrenal glands, from which they derive their name. The adrenal glands and central nervous system maintain high levels of vitamin C by means of special cellular pumps, which absorb the vitamin when the body is deficient.

Vitamin C is also needed for synthesis of carnitine, a small molecule involved in transporting fat (lipids) to mitochondria, the "furnaces" of the body's cells that burn nutrients to produce energy.[1] The energy provided is used either to power the cells' activities or to provide antioxidant electrons that prevent harmful oxidation.

Vitamin C is involved in breaking down cholesterol to form bile acids. This may have implications for people wishing to lower their cholesterol levels. While the role of cholesterol in causing cardiovascular disease is generally overstated, vitamin C's action on cholesterol levels suggests that higher levels may lower the risk of gallstones.[2]

Vitamin C is widely known as an antioxidant, a substance that fights free radicals, which can damage tissues and cause illness. As the principal water-soluble antioxidant in the diet, vitamin C is essential to health. A shortage of vitamin C results in free radical damage to essential molecules in the body. The molecules affected include DNA (deoxyribonucleic acid) and RNA (ribonucleic acid), proteins, lipids (fats), and carbohydrates. Mitochondria, chemical toxins from smoking, and x-rays are examples of sources of damaging free radicals and oxidation.

The importance of vitamin C in preventing free radical damage, aging, and oxidation is sometimes understated. An adequate supply of vitamin C enables the regeneration of vitamin E and other antioxidants in the body. The main water-soluble antioxidant generated within our cells is called glutathione, a small protein molecule (tripeptide of the amino acids glutamic acid, cysteine, and glycine) that plays a central role in protecting our cells from oxidation damage.[3] Since it is typically present in ten times the concentration of vitamin C, it has often been considered to play a more important role. However, the functions of vitamin C and glutathione are linked.

In animals that make their own vitamin C, those deprived of glutathione compensate by synthesizing additional vitamin C. Feeding animals vitamin C can increase their glutathione levels and high levels of glutathione can prevent loss of vitamin C. In guinea pigs and newborn rats, which are unable to synthesize ascorbate, glutathione deficiency is lethal. However, death can be prevented in such animals by giving high doses of ascorbate.[4] Similarly, the onset of scurvy in guinea pigs fed an ascorbate-deficient diet can be delayed by giving glutathione monoethyl ester, a glutathione delivery agent.[5] A primary role for glutathione is to recycle oxidized vitamin C so it can continue to function as an antioxidant. Vitamin C is required for the antioxidant functioning of glutathione, even when glutathione is present in a vastly greater concentration.[6] This relationship between antioxidants suggests that a high intake of vitamin C is crucial for preventing the oxidation damage associated with disease and aging.

The Vitamin C Muddle

Just about everything doctors have been telling us about vitamin C is wrong. Current medical opinion says that people can gain all their vitamin requirements from a healthy diet. We are told to make sure we get five, or perhaps even nine, helpings of fruits and vegetables each day, and that we do not need dietary supplements. Eating fruits and vegetables will help prevent heart disease and cancer. However, people have not adopted this change in diet. In a survey of 4,278 people in the United Kingdom, two-thirds stated that they did not eat the recommended portions of fruits and vegetables.[7] In Northern Ireland, only 17 percent of people reported eating five helpings each day. It is not surprising that people are unwilling to accept government recommendations, considering the lack of supporting evidence and the inconsistencies in the advice.

Inuit Indians ate a high-protein, high-fat diet. Traditional Eskimos, in an environment of stark landscapes shaped by glacial temperatures, lived on a diet with little plant food and no farm or dairy products. Inuits mostly subsisted on simple hunting and fishing. Coastal Indians exploited the sea, while those further inland took advantage of caribou, including predigested vegetation in the animals' stomachs consisting of mosses, lichens, and the available tundra plants. But Inuits were not subject to high levels of heart disease, despite this diet high in saturated fat and low in fruits and vegetables. Similarly, people on the Atkins diet have not had the suggested increased risk of heart disease. These diets are hardly balanced in the conventional sense and do not comprise the mix of grains, fruits, vegetables, meat, eggs, and dairy in the government-recommended food pyramids. Such diets conventionally should not be adequate. While Inuits must eat a few milligrams of vitamin C to prevent acute scurvy, people are expected to succumb rapidly to ill health on a diet of little but fat and animal protein—at least that's what the so-called experts have been telling us.

Inuits retain reasonable health on an apparently poor diet.[8] The Inuit and Atkins diets have something in common that provides adequacy while being less than optimal for health. The Inuit diet modifies the antioxidant profile and may reduce free radical damage and the need for high levels of vitamin C.[9] They both contain a relatively high ratio of vitamin C to sugar. While the intake of vitamin C is low in the Inuit diet, the drop in carbohydrates is far larger. A typical Western diet may include 500 grams of carbohydrate each day but less than 50 milligrams (mg) of vitamin C. Importantly, sugar prevents the absorption of vitamin C into cells. While the Inuits have a lower intake of vitamin C, they use the molecule more efficiently, as the competition with sugars and particularly glucose is correspondingly lower. The low-carbohydrate Inuit diet partly compensates for a low vitamin C intake.

The principal benefit of fruits and vegetables is an increased intake of antioxidants, particularly vitamin C. This book explains why eating more vegetables, while good advice, will not provide the benefits of vitamin C supplementation. Some doctors claim that high-dose vitamin C acts as a powerful anti-infective agent, potentially to eradicate heart disease and to prevent or treat cancer. No one claims that eating a few additional vegetables will provide the massive benefits ascribed to vitamin C.

Straight from the Horse's Mouth

The controversy over vitamin C became well-known when Nobel Prize–winning chemist Linus Pauling, Ph.D., advocated megadoses to prevent and treat diseases, such as the common cold. Dr. Pauling suggested that people need doses 100 times greater than those recommended by doctors and other nutritional experts. The medical profession's response was a devastating attack on Dr. Pauling's scientific competence, some even labeling him a "quack." After Dr. Pauling's death in 1994, the medical establishment alleged they had shown that he was wrong and that people needed only small amounts of vitamin C. If people consumed more, they suggested, it would not be absorbed and so could not have the health effects claimed by Dr. Pauling and others. As we shall see, recent scientific evidence does not support this position.

Historically, vitamins were considered micronutrients and thought to be essential to good health. Without these, a person could become sick or might even die. A micronutrient is a substance, such as a vitamin or mineral, needed in minute amounts for the proper growth and metabolism of a living organism. By definition, larger amounts of micronutrients are inessential and might even be toxic.

Vitamin C was named before the substance that prevents its associated deficiency disease, scurvy, was discovered and isolated. This was premature, as its properties could not be determined before its chemical identity. The designation "vitamin C" presupposes that only small amounts of the substance are needed. When Albert Szent-Györgyi, M.D., Ph.D., first isolated ascorbic acid and identified it as vitamin C, in the period from 1927 to 1933, he was aware that this preconception could prejudice subsequent scientific investigation. From the start, Dr. Szent-Györgyi suspected that, for optimal health, people might need gram levels of vitamin C.

As other vitamins were isolated and investigated, the amounts needed to prevent acute disease appeared to be small, so the idea of vitamins as micronutrients became nutritional dogma. Since then, scientific opinion on most vitamins has diverged into two camps. The first has governmental and official support, largely for historical reasons. This official grouping considers that the intake of vitamins should be just enough to prevent acute deficiency symptoms, such as scurvy. According to the conventional view, intakes above this minimum level are considered unnecessary and may have some theoretical dangers. For vitamin C, these dangers are currently unsupported by evidence.

A second set of scientists and physicians, who we call the orthomolecular group, take the view that the evidence is incomplete. *Orthomolecular* is a word coined by Linus Pauling to describe the use of nutrients and normal ("ortho") constituents of the body in optimum amounts as the primary treatment. Thus, optimal health may require more than the minimum intake. Scientists in this group consider that the evidence on the health effects of vitamin and nutrient intake is woefully inadequate—in other words, we do not have the data to determine optimal intakes. If the orthomolecular scientists are correct, optimal nutrition might prevent much chronic human disease.

Surprisingly, for most vitamins and minerals, the difference between conventional and orthomolecular recommendations is not large. The government Recommended Dietary Allowance (RDA) for vitamin E is 22 International Units (IU) per day, while orthomolecular-oriented physicians typically recommend higher levels, in the range 100–1,000 IU per day (5–50 times the RDA). By comparison, the corresponding discrepancy for vitamin C is huge. The RDA for vitamin C in the United States is 90 mg per day for an adult male, whereas scientists such as Dr. Pauling have recommended values of 2–20 grams (2,000–20,000 mg) per day. This difference is even greater for people who are ill. The official position is that levels of vitamin C higher than the 90 mg are not beneficial in illness. However, physicians such as Robert F. Cathcart III, a pioneering vitamin C researcher, have been using doses of up to 200 grams (200,000 mg) per day to treat disease, an intake over 2,000 times the RDA.

There is a pertinent story attributed to Francis Bacon (1561–1626), a leading figure in natural philosophy who worked in the transitional period between the Renaissance and the early modern era.[10] In 1432, some friars had a quarrel about the number of teeth in a horse's mouth. The argument raged for thirteen days, as the scholars consulted ancient books and manuscripts in an effort to obtain a definitive answer. Then, on the fourteenth day, a young friar asked innocently if he should find a horse and look inside its mouth. With a mighty uproar, the others attacked him and cast him out. Clearly, Satan had tempted the neophyte to declare unholy ways of finding the truth, contrary to the teaching of the fathers!

Bacon's story sounds quaint in our current technological age. Unfortunately, the friars' way of hiding from reality, by stipulating how people should search for the truth, is prevalent in modern medicine. As the story of vitamin C unfolds, this simple nutrient will expose modern medicine as a craft, dominated by institutional authorities, rather than a scientific discipline. For example, clinical trials have used unscientific myths about placebo function to negate nutritional effects. Medical traditionalists have misrepresented low doses of vitamin C as corresponding to the massive doses claimed to be effective. Mainstream medicine sidelines and ignores the clinical observations on high-dose vitamin C to the detriment of people's health.

A Matter of Survival

Although vitamin C is essential to life, most animals do not need to consume it because they manufacture it within their bodies. However, some animals, including humans, have lost the ability to synthesize vitamin C. They have become, in effect, ascorbate mutants, reliant on vitamin C in their diet. Without it, they die—deficiency in humans, apes, and guinea pigs causes a fatal disease, scurvy.

About 40 million years ago, the ancestors of human beings were small, furry mammals. One such creature lost the gene for an enzyme necessary to synthesize ascorbic acid, perhaps because of a radiation-induced genetic mutation.[11] Offspring of this mutant were consequently unable to make vitamin C. Presumably, they were largely vegetarian, consuming a diet rich in ascorbic acid, so loss of the enzyme was not catastrophic.

Evolutionary fitness is the ability of an organism to leave viable offspring. Surprisingly, loss of the gene for making vitamin C did not have a hugely detrimental effect on the evolutionary fitness and survival of our ancestors. We know this because, otherwise, animal species with this mutation would have died out, and they did not. It is probable that some animals, including humans, gained an evolutionary advantage by losing the gene for vitamin C.

Humans are not the only creatures who need to consume vitamin C. Others include guinea pigs, apes, some bats, and several bird species. These animals have all evolved successfully, surviving in the struggle for existence for millions of years. If the ability to manufacture vitamin C was lost only once during evolution, we might conclude it was an interesting oddity. However, on the tree of life, birds and mammals diverged much earlier than the time our ancestors lost the gene. Birds appear to have originated from reptiles, in the Upper Jurassic and Lower Cretaceous periods (about 150 million years ago). Mammals evolved from reptiles much earlier, in the Carboniferous and Permian periods (about 250–350 million years ago). This suggests that birds and mammals lost their genes for making vitamin C separately and independently.

In humans, lack of vitamin C causes scurvy, which leads to bleeding and bruising throughout the body. Gums swell, teeth fall out, and, within a few months, the sufferer dies a horrible death. On early sea voyages, scurvy killed many sailors. Strangely, some people were more resistant to the disease than others, which might indicate that a few people retain some biochemical ability to make the vitamin or sustain its levels in the body. Fortunately, even a few milligrams of vitamin C each day will prevent acute scurvy. We might wonder why early humans did not die of scurvy and become extinct. However, herbivorous animals, including apes, live largely on a diet of vegetables; their vitamin C intake is high. By studying the diet of the great apes, Linus Pauling estimated that early humans probably had an intake of between 2.5 and 9 grams of vitamin C a day.[12] If an animal ate a diet with plenty of vitamin C, loss of the gene to make it would not have caused loss of evolutionary fitness. Consequently, we can reasonably assume that our early ancestors were largely vegetarian.

Evolutionary success also depends on reproduction. Provided the young could consume enough vitamin C to prevent acute scurvy, absence of the gene might not have lowered the early humans' evolutionary fitness. There would have to be sufficient vitamin C to prevent disease and maintain fitness levels throughout the period of conceiving and bringing up children.

In times of plenty, loss of the vitamin C gene may have had only a marginal effect. Indeed, vegetarian animals without the gene might have a slight energetic advantage, as they did not need to manufacture the substance internally. Animals with the gene and mutants that had lost it could have coexisted for long periods in the same population. However, when food supplies became short, those that did not waste vital energy making vitamin C may have had a survival advantage. In the words of

Dr. Cathcart, the mutants could "out starve" those with the gene. During periods of severe evolutionary stress, animals without the vitamin C gene could predominate to the point that those with the gene became extinct.

An Evolutionary Advantage

Several lines of evidence suggest that the human population has crashed in the past. For many species, evolutionary bottlenecks are surprisingly common because a species exists for only as long as it can compete for its place in the ecosystem. Most species that have existed on earth are already extinct. A typical species has a lifetime of about 10 million years.[13] Current evidence suggests humans almost became extinct about 150,000 years ago. Genetic studies suggest that all humans arose from a small population in Africa only 150,000 to 200,000 years ago.[14] A creative interpretation of the scientific facts traces all human life back to a single woman, living about 150,000 years ago in East Africa, the area that now encompasses Ethiopia, Kenya, and Tanzania. "Mitochondrial Eve," as she is known, is the most recent common female, or matrilineal, ancestor of all humans.[15]

To understand the significance of Mitochondrial Eve, remember that human cells contain small particles called mitochondria that hold the biochemical machinery to supply us with energy. Mitochondria have their own genetic material (DNA), which is transferred to children by way of the mother's egg (ovum).[16] The male sperm is much smaller than the ovum and does not supply mitochondria to the fetus. Scientists have shown that all humans contain mitochondrial DNA originating from a single individual. This Eve did not live alone but probably dwelt in a small village or community, where her children had some evolutionary advantage over others in the tribe.

There is a corresponding common male ancestor, called "Y-chromosomal Adam," who lived 60,000 to 90,000 years ago. Chromosomes are packages of genes that transfer DNA to the cells of the offspring. Male children get a Y chromosome from their father, which pairs up with an X chromosome from the mother, creating the XY pair that determines the male sex. Females get one X chromosome from each parent, forming an XX pair. Scientists have traced mutations in the Y chromosome back in time to identify Y-chromosomal Adam. Unlike the biblical Adam, Y-chromosomal

Adam lived many tens of thousands of years after Mitochondrial Eve. Our Adam and Eve should not be considered as scientific facts, but as stories to illustrate one possible interpretation of the available evidence.

A possible explanation for Y-chromosomal Adam is a super-volcanic event that occurred 70,000 to 75,000 years ago at Lake Toba in Indonesia, which might have devastated the human population.[17] Humans could have been reduced to a few thousand breeding pairs, creating a bottleneck in human evolution. The geological event was perhaps thousands of times greater in magnitude than the 1980 eruption of Mount St. Helens and may have lowered the global temperature for several years, potentially triggering an ice age. It is possible that Y-chromosomal Adam was simply the most successful survivor of the Toba super-volcanic catastrophe.

This narrative illustrates how selection pressures on humans can be severe. If loss of the vitamin C gene provided increased ability to survive periods of starvation, it may even have secured the ultimate survival of the human race. It is possible to explain our Mitochondrial Eve by assuming that a mutation in her mitochondrial DNA gave her a large advantage over other humans. In this case, people with Eve's mitochondria would have increased in the population and could have eventually replaced all other forms. We could explain Y-chromosomal Adam in a similar way.

Unlike apes and many other mammals, humans have little genetic diversity; this may have been caused by population bottlenecks.[18] Any gene that is represented in only a small number of individuals is at risk of elimination. There have been many times when lack of the gene for vitamin C could have bestowed an evolutionary advantage. Population bottlenecks may have ensured that individuals without the gene came to dominate. We carry the consequences of this evolutionary accident in our genes.

Cost of the Lost Gene

Despite this evolutionary benefit, the loss of the gene for vitamin C may have left older people facing severe deficits and disease. Once an animal has reproduced, evolutionary selection is less effective. In modern humans and some animal groups, grandparents may be involved in raising the young, but, in evolutionary terms, this is a secondary factor. In the wild, older animals can be rare and extended family groups are the exception. The loss of the gene for vitamin C could lead to numerous problems, including arthritis, cardiovascular disease, cancer, and decreased immune response. However, death of an animal that has completed its reproductive phase does not prevent its successful offspring from forming the next generation. Provided these chronic diseases occurred later in life, their effect on evolutionary fitness would be small. In evolutionary terms, it does not matter if an old guinea pig suffers, provided it has left a large number of healthy young offspring.

Thus, human evolution may have provided the ability to survive periods of food shortage, but at the expense of chronic disease. Such disease would only be an issue if the intake of vitamin C in the diet were insufficient for long-term needs. We know little about our mammalian ancestors at the time the vitamin C gene was lost. Forty million years ago is shortly after the dinosaurs became extinct and we have only a sparse record of fossilized bones from that era. More importantly, we have little information about the diet of our ancestors.

The typical diet of modern humans does not consist predominantly of vitamin C–rich vegetables. Although people live reasonably long lives with this limited intake, they increasingly suffer degenerative diseases and a lower quality of life. This unnecessary suffering might not happen if the lost gene were still present. Our inability to make our own ascorbate means that each newborn baby comes factory-equipped with, if not an inborn vitamin C deficiency, a vitamin C dependency.

The Health Benefits of Vitamin C

The genuine vitamin C story has become clearer over recent years, as claims for unique health benefits of vitamin C are consistent with the available evidence. There is little scientific support for the idea that low (RDA level) doses of ascorbate are optimal for humans. Antioxidants like vitamin C are essential for life because disease processes almost invariably involve free radical attack, which antioxidant defenses can counteract.

People visiting a physician expect to receive clear, unbiased information about what ails them and its treatments. More importantly, they need to know what they can do to prevent disease. Patients would like to have the information necessary to make informed choices, but in many cases, this information is not provided, and even doctors are often unable to evaluate the information they need to make decisions that are optimal for patients' interests.[19] People often disregard the advice of conventional experts and supplement their diet with gram-level doses of vitamin C and other antioxidants. Perhaps surprisingly, diverse groups of independent individuals can often produce more accurate solutions than those obtained by selected committees of experts.[20] Thus, this popular decision could be a sign that medicine has gone astray and is refusing, unable, or unwilling, to respond rationally to the evidence.

Gram-level doses of vitamin C may prevent many diseases, but much higher doses are required for treatment of illness. The massive doses needed for therapy are often greeted with disbelief. When we inform doctors that 50–100 grams (50,000–100,000 mg) of vitamin C per day may be required to treat a common cold, their skepticism is transferred from the efficacy of the treatment to the size of the dose. Most clinical studies have considered doses of a single gram. A dose 100 times larger has very different properties.

One reason for the vitamin C controversy is contradictory clinical results from trials that used inadequate doses, doses that are 100 times too small and have consistently broken the basic rules of pharmacology.[21] For an analogy, imagine a study in which 20,000 fertile young women are placed on the contraceptive pill to prevent pregnancy. The researchers want to show the pill has no effect, so they give one pill a month, instead of one a day, as designed. Control subjects take one sugar pill (placebo) per month. Now, suppose the results of this five-year trial indicate that, when taking a contraceptive pill once a month, the women became pregnant at the same rate as those on the sugar pill. No reasonable person would accept the claim that "the trial shows the pill does not prevent pregnancy." You cannot expect a daily pill given monthly to have the same effect as the daily dose. However, this methodology is equivalent to studies of "high-dose" vitamin C, which have purported to show it is ineffective.

An optimal intake of vitamin C is the amount that prevents disease while minimizing the potential risk. It is a huge assumption to think that an intake to prevent acute scurvy will be adequate to prevent other diseases. Furthermore, there is substantial evidence that the intake of vitamin C needed to prevent chronic illness is much greater than the RDA. Unfortunately, direct studies on chronic disease and high-dose vitamin C intakes have not been undertaken, so we have to base our conclusions on an insufficient knowledge base. Typically, prospective studies provide the most direct information. In a prospective study, vitamin C intake is estimated in large numbers of subjects, who are then tracked over time to see if they develop specific chronic diseases. Such studies are expensive and often imprecise. For example, the vitamin intake may be estimated by a questionnaire and approximated from typical proportions found in particular food items. People's diets may change with time and content tables do not take account of specific items—fresh, organic carrots contain more vitamin C than those found in cans, for example. To get an accurate estimate of the optimal intake, it would be necessary for these studies to include intakes of vitamin C ranging from 50 mg up to at least 10,000 mg per day, and this has not been done. Some researchers suggest strangely that vitamin C from food is somehow more effective than the same molecule contained in supplements. However, an alternative explanation is that the methods used to estimate vitamin C intake from food have limited accuracy. Another possible explanation relates to the fact that we eat several times a day and vitamin C is released from food more gradually than from supplements.[22]

Scurvy

Many people connect the word *scurvy* with history lessons rather than modern day health. The British Admiralty finally, after a delay of fifty years, enacted James Lind's 1747 finding that consumption of citrus fruit could prevent scurvy. In the intervening period, thousands of sailors died. Unfortunately for them, the cost of providing citrus fruit was greater than the cost of a press gang. Then, as now, economic considerations often took priority over science or people's well-being.

People with acute scurvy eventually suffer bruising, bleeding into their joints causing swelling and severe pain, and loss of hair and teeth. These symptoms are, as we have explained, a result of collagen shortage. Earlier onset symptoms include fatigue, arising from the reduced ability to make carnitine, and susceptibility to stress because of lower levels of adrenaline and noradrenaline.

In developed countries, acute scurvy is rare, as consuming a few milligrams of vitamin C daily prevents the illness, while outbreaks of scurvy are more frequent in the Third World. However, even in developed areas, people with chronic illness, the infirm, elderly, and children can be at risk, and low blood levels of vitamin C are common.[23] Chronic scurvy may arise if a person has sufficient vitamin C intake to prevent a painful death in the short-term, but not enough to keep them healthy.

Preventing Heart Disease and Stroke

Many prospective studies indicate that low intakes of vitamin C are associated with an increased risk of cardiovascular disease. Despite such studies not including an investigation of higher intakes, it was assumed wrongly that approximately 100 mg of vitamin C per day gives a maximum risk reduction. The first National Health and Nutrition Examination Study (NHANES I) estimated that the risk of death from cardiovascular diseases was 25 percent lower in women and 42 percent lower in men who supplemented with vitamin C.[24] The average intake of supplemental vitamin C was 300 mg per day.[25]

A review of nine studies, covering 290,000 adults, found that those who supplemented with more than 700 mg of vitamin C per day had a 25 percent lower risk of heart disease. These subjects had apparently healthy cardiovascular systems at the start of the ten-year study.[26] A study of over 85,000 female nurses over a period of sixteen years found that higher vitamin C intakes helped prevent heart disease.[27] Once again, high intakes of vitamin C from supplements (average of 359 mg per day) were linked to a 27–28 percent reduction in risk of heart disease. Notably, nurses who did not take supplements did not benefit from this risk reduction.

Similar results have been obtained with vitamin C and stroke. One study covered a twenty-year observation period documenting 196 cases of stroke (including 109 infarctions and 54 hemorrhages). The subjects with the highest vitamin C blood levels had a 29 percent lower risk of stroke than those with the lowest levels.[28] This study of a Japanese rural community followed 880 men and 1,241 women aged forty years and older who were initially free of stroke when examined in 1977. Not surprisingly, those people who ate vegetables nearly every day had a lower risk of stroke than those who ate them two days a week or less. Blood plasma levels of vitamin C increased with fruit and vegetable intakes. While it is possible that some other component of the fruit and vegetable intake contributed to the reported benefit, there is no evidence to support this suggestion. There is also no evidence that people who ate fruits and vegetables may have benefited from associated behaviors or lifestyle. A more scientific approach is to note that even the plasma levels in this study correspond to deficiency and were below the well-nourished baseline. One may wonder how low the incidence of stroke could have been had these subjects been provided with appropriate vitamin C supplementation.

As might be expected from such a blunt experimental procedure, some prospective epidemiological studies have not revealed a lower risk of cardiovascular disease with vitamin C supplement use.[29] Taken as a whole, however, these results suggest that in order to lower heart attack risk, vitamin C intakes may need to be high enough to maintain the body pool.[30] It is also possible that much higher intakes of vitamin C could effectively eradicate heart disease from the population.

Preventing Cancer

People generally accept that eating fruits and vegetables reduces the risk of many types of cancer.[31] Vegetables contain a large number of phytonutrients and other cancer-preventing substances, so it is not obvious how much of the benefit might be a result of increased vitamin C intake.

Higher daily intakes of vitamin C are associated with a reduced risk of cancer in many organs, including the mouth, neck, lungs, and the digestive tract (esophagus, stomach, and colon). In one study, men with an intake of more than 83 mg of vitamin C daily had a 64 percent lower risk of lung cancer compared with those with an intake of less than 63 mg per day. This study followed 870 people over twenty-five years.[32] Studies have linked an increased vitamin C intake with a lower risk of stomach cancer. The ulcer-forming bacterium *Helicobacter pylori* is associated with increased risk of stomach cancer. Since this bacterium decreases the amount of vitamin C in stomach secretions, supplementation has been suggested as an adjunct to antibiotic therapy for ulcers.[33]

Most large surveys have found little association between breast cancer and the low intakes of vitamin C that are typically studied. However, in one study, overweight women with an average vitamin C intake of 110 mg each day were found to have a 39 percent lower risk of breast cancer compared to similar women with an intake of 31 mg a day.[34] The Nurses' Health Study also suggests an association between low levels of vitamin C and breast cancer. A 63 percent lower risk of breast cancer was found in premenopausal women with an average intake of 205 mg of vitamin C per day compared with similar women who consumed an average of 70 mg each day.[35] These subjects had a family history of breast cancer. Unfortunately, once again, data on higher intakes of vitamin C (in the range 1,000 to 10,000 mg) are not available.

Viral Illnesses

Reported results of treatment with massive doses of vitamin C are almost without parallel in medical history. A classic example is the study by Frederick R. Klenner, M.D., on polio. Around 1950, Dr. Klenner claimed that he could cure polio in a few days using vitamin C. This was at a time before polio vaccination and often patients were paralyzed or died, but Dr. Klenner reported that none of his patients died or suffered paralysis.

A research group led by Dr. Jonathan Gould in the 1950s conducted a placebo-controlled trial of vitamin C as a treatment for polio.[36] About seventy children were treated in the study; half the children were given vitamin C and the remainder a placebo. All the children given vitamin C recovered. However, in the placebo group, approximately 20 percent had residual impairment. Dr. Gould did not report his conclusions because the Salk vaccine for polio had just been announced and, at that time, there was great hope and expectancy for the benefits of vaccination. However, if the report was correct, these results with vitamin C are more fundamental.

Vitamin C may act as a general "antibiotic" against all forms of viral disease. People still die of polio and many cases have occurred because of the use of live polio vaccination.[37] Researchers have not found any comparable treatment for the unfortunate individuals who contract polio or other viral diseases each year. Astoundingly, similar claims by reputable physicians for vitamin C treatment of a wide range of viral illnesses continued over the following half century without being subject to clinical testing.

Heavy Metal Toxicity

Heavy metal toxicity is a continuing problem. Lead has been a problem for humanity for thousands of years and, for a time, was thought to be responsible for the fall of the Roman Empire. One idea was that the toxic properties of lead pipes caused widespread mental deficits. It is more likely that such effects were small, but produced a loss of vigor and fitness relative to other competing civilizations.[38] Lead pipes had been used for several centuries before the fall of Rome and continued to be used in England, for example, until they were gradually phased out in the twentieth century. The toxic effect was not strong enough to prevent the burst of intellectual activity leading to and propelling the Industrial Revolution.

Recent problems of heavy metal poisoning involve lead from car exhaust, aluminum in water, and mercury in fillings.[39] We will use lead poisoning as an example of the protective role of vitamin C. This poisoning is occasionally seen in pregnant women, in whom it can induce abnormal growth and development of the fetus. Children chronically exposed to lead suffer behavioral problems and learning disabilities. In adults, lead toxicity can produce high blood pressure and kidney damage. In older men, higher blood vitamin C levels are associated with lower lead concentrations in the body. A study of lead levels in 747 elderly men showed that oral vitamin C intakes of less than 109 mg per day were linked to higher lead in blood and bone than those consuming 339 mg or more each day.[40] This result was supported by a study of 19,578 people, which indicated that higher serum vitamin C levels were linked with significantly lower blood lead concentrations.[41]

The response of blood lead levels to moderate intakes of vitamin C can occur in a matter of weeks. A placebo-controlled study of the effects of vitamin C supplementation (1,000 mg daily) on blood lead concentrations in 75 adult male smokers measured significant reductions (81 percent) in lead levels within a month.[42] Lower intakes (200 mg per day) did not affect blood lead concentrations.

Cataracts

Considering its role in protection from free radical damage, vitamin C might be predicted to prevent cataracts, one of the leading causes of visual impairment.[43] Cataracts arise for a number of reasons, including long-term ultraviolet (UV) light exposure and other ionizing radiation. They are also associated with high glucose levels in diabetics, and increase in frequency and severity with age. The primary effect of cataracts is to denature (deform) certain proteins called crystallins in the lens of the eye.

More severe cataracts are linked with low vitamin C levels in the eye. Unsurprisingly, therefore, increased blood plasma levels of vitamin C are also associated with decreased severity of cataracts.[44] Increased vitamin C intake associates with lower cataracts in some but not all studies, presumably because the doses were not frequent enough to consistently raise blood and eye levels.[45] A trial of antioxidant supplementation, including vitamin C (500 mg), vitamin E (400 IU), and beta-carotene (15 mg), in 4,629 adults over six years found no effect on the development and progression of cataracts.[46] Some possible reasons for this lack of effect are that the vitamin C dose was small and some participants were given copper, which interacts with vitamin C, causing oxidation. Also, the form of vitamin E used was synthetic dl-alpha-tocopherol, which is often used in studies but is less biologically active than natural, mixed tocotrienols and tocopherols.

At some stage, almost every chronic disease has been related to an insufficient intake of vitamin C. The scientific evidence available is sparse and it may take centuries to determine which chronic illnesses are related to a shortage of vitamin C. In the meantime, the optimal amount of vitamin C is a matter of continued debate. It is time that medical scientists realized that attacking and denigrating vitamin C and other nutritional therapies can no longer be tolerated. An open, scientific approach to vitamin C and other nutrients could offer major benefits to humanity.

CHAPTER 2

The Pioneers of Vitamin C Research

*"The conventional view serves to protect us
from the painful job of thinking."*
—JOHN KENNETH GALBRAITH

"Eat your fruits! Eat your greens! They are full of goodness," our grandmothers used to say. The advice was excellent, as these foods include essential vitamins that, together with minerals and phytonutrients, help prevent disease and keep us healthy. Current nutritional advice to eat between five and nine helpings of fruit and vegetables is consistent with our grandmothers' advice, but does not recognize that the science of nutrition has made rapid advances in recent decades. We can now isolate and identify the beneficial substances in food.

The Discovery of Vitamin C

The first vitamins were identified at the beginning of the twentieth century. Christiaan Eijkman and his collaborator, Gerrit Grijns, had shown that rice bran contained small amounts of a substance that prevents disease in chickens. Then, in 1906, British biochemist Sir Frederick Hopkins fed rats a diet of artificial milk, made from protein, fat, carbohydrates, and mineral salts. He found that they did not grow as expected. However, adding a little cow's milk to their diet allowed the rats to develop rapidly. In order to grow, the rats clearly needed some additional substance in the milk.

In 1912, Dr. Hopkins and Casimir Funk proposed that the absence of sufficient amounts of certain substances in food causes disease. Their "vitamin hypothesis" suggested the existence of four vitamins that provided protection against four diseases:

- Vitamin B$_1$, which prevents beriberi

- Vitamin B$_3$, which prevents pellagra

- Vitamin D, which prevents rickets

- Vitamin C, which prevents scurvy

Drs. Eijkman and Hopkins shared the 1929 Nobel Prize for the discovery that vitamins are essential to maintain health.

When the anti-scurvy substance was given the name vitamin C, no one knew what it was. They knew that it was found in fruit, because pioneers such as James Lind had shown in the eighteenth century that citrus fruit could cure scurvy in sailors. However, there must be a specific chemical in fruit and vegetables preventing and healing scurvy for the vitamin C hypothesis to be correct. By 1928, Albert Szent-Györgyi, M.D., Ph.D., a Hungarian biochemist working in Cambridge, had isolated a strong antioxidant, a white powder found in fruit and vegetables. He realized that he had found the elusive vitamin C, for which he was awarded the 1937 Nobel Prize in medicine. Dr. Szent-Györgyi consistently suggested that people might need gram-level intakes of vitamin C for good health, but his views were in the minority.

Vitamins were defined as micronutrients and this paradigm has been applied to ascorbate. However, the idea that ascorbate is different and people need massive intakes of vitamin C existed at the time ascorbic acid was first identified and isolated. Since then, the views have polarized and doctors who study our need for large intakes of vitamin C have been marginalized. For decades, pioneering doctors have investigated the clinical effects of massive doses of vitamin C. Their reports of remarkable clinical benefits have been replicated many times and their contributions have become part of the foundations of orthomolecular medicine.

Irwin Stone

Irwin Stone, Ph.D. (1907–1984), was one of the earliest scientists to realize vitamin C's potential. Dr. Stone was an industrial chemist who began considering its use as a food preservative before the substance changed his life. Dr. Stone was educated as a biochemist and chemical engineer in New York. From 1924 to 1934, he worked at the Pease Laboratories, initially as an assistant bacteriologist before eventually being promoted to chief chemist.[1] He followed this by setting up and directing an early biochemistry laboratory for the Wallerstein Company. Dr. Stone used vitamin C to prevent oxidation in food, a purpose for which it is still commonly employed. He gained the first patents on industrial applications of ascorbic acid as a food preservative and antioxidant, eventually publishing over 120 scientific articles and obtaining twenty-six U.S. patents.

He became convinced that high intakes of vitamin C would be greatly beneficial to health. In the 1930s, soon after it first became commercially available, Dr. Stone began supplementing his diet with large amounts of vitamin C. He proposed that humans had inherited a genetic trait to need, but not manufacture, ascorbic acid.[2] This innate dependency may be satisfied from our diets, but not easily.[3] According to Dr. Stone, the present recommendations for vitamin C are more than 100 times less than what we really need, based on the amount produced endogenously each day by other mammals.[4] He repeatedly stated that ignoring this fact would prove fatal.[5]

A prime example of a disease attributed to vitamin C deficiency is Sudden Infant Death Syndrome (SIDS). Two Australian doctors, Archie Kalokerinos and Glen Dettman, showed that SIDS could be a manifestation of infantile scurvy. Mothers depend solely on their diet for vitamin C, so if they are deficient, children are born with chronic, subclinical scurvy. If they are correct, increasing the infant's intake of vitamin C would prevent SIDS.[6] Dr. Stone suggests that up to 10,000 babies a year die of SIDS unnecessarily. Unfortunately, the medical establishment, complacent with the idea that scurvy is a disease of the past, has not followed up on these clinical observations.

Dr. Stone's work on vitamin C continued and by the late 1950s he had reached the conclusion that scurvy was far more widespread than realized. Furthermore, vitamin C did not have the expected properties of a micronutrient, as the body needs larger amounts.[7] In his view, ascorbic acid was not a vitamin at all, but an essential dietary factor needed in much larger quantities than a micronutrient.[8] Animals make large amounts of ascorbic acid in their livers or kidneys. Dr. Stone believed that people needed much larger amounts of vitamin C than the medical establishment recommended.[9]

In April 1966, Dr. Stone met Linus Pauling, Ph.D., and told him his ideas about vitamin C.[10] Dr. Pauling, then in his mid-sixties, said that he wished he might live another twenty-five years, as science was advancing rapidly and he would like to be around to follow developments. Dr. Stone suggested he could achieve his goal by taking megadoses of vitamin C. Dr. Pauling, convinced by the arguments, embarked on a regimen of high-dose vitamin C and went on to live the claimed twenty-five years, and a few more.[11]

Dr. Stone had by that time assembled a large collection of vitamin C papers. Notably, he hated the term "vitamin C" and used its alternative chemical names, ascorbic acid or ascorbate. Dr. Stone appears to have originated the word *megavitamin* and used the word *hypoascorbemia* to describe a subclinical deficiency of vitamin C.[12] He argued that scurvy was not a deficiency disease, but a metabolic error. In 1971, when he retired, he dedicated the rest of his life to studying and making people aware of the need for daily gram-level consumption of vitamin C.

In 1972, Dr. Stone published fifty years' worth of research and observation in his book, *The Healing Factor: Vitamin C Against Disease*. This contained a summarized account of successful vitamin C treatments for infections (bacterial and viral), allergies, asthma, poisoning, ulcers, the effects of smoking, and eye diseases, including glaucoma. He also described the treatment of cancer, heart disease, diabetes, fractures, bladder and kidney diseases, tetanus, shock, wounds, and pregnancy complications. Despite a statement by the National Health Federation that the book may be "the most important book on health ever written," conventional medicine largely ignored it.

Vitamin C Saved His Life

The high doses of vitamin C that Dr. Stone was taking may even have saved his life. Vitamin C and other antioxidants can reduce the stress associated with trauma,[13] and for Dr. Stone, this action of vitamin C was critical in his recovery from a severe road accident. He tells the story himself:

> Outside of Rapid City, South Dakota, we had a very serious automobile accident when a drunk driving on the wrong side of the road drove her car at 80 miles an hour into a head-on collision with ours. Both my wife and I were seriously injured and the only reason we survived was the fact that we had been regularly taking daily megadoses of ascorbate for decades. We never went into the deep shock that kills most accident victims and I was able to experimentally verify

ascorbate's great healing power and survival value by taking about 50 to 60 grams a day of ascorbate during our hospitalization. . . . I went through five serious operations without any surgical shock and my multiple bone injuries healed so fast that we were able to leave the hospital in less than three months, take a 2,000-mile train trip home, and I was back at work running my lab in two months more. . . . My larynx was damaged by part of the steering wheel inflicting a deep throat wound, and the doctors despaired that I would ever talk again. With the help of megascorbics, this problem slowly resolved and I was able to assume the public speaking duties.[14]

There is some understatement in Dr. Stone's account. His son, Steve, a retired patent attorney, adds that his parents' car was hit with such force that all of his father's limbs, except his right arm, were broken and he had massive internal injuries. Dr. Stone needed an emergency tracheotomy, and by the time he reached the hospital he had lost a lot of blood, yet he never went into shock. They were both in the hospital from May until August. As soon as he could communicate, Dr. Stone insisted on having vitamin C supplements and convinced those caring for him that it was the reason he survived.[15]

A Megavitamin Pioneer

Linus Pauling was a staunch supporter of Dr. Stone's work, as was Dr. Szent-Györgyi. In 1982, Dr. Stone wrote to Dr. Szent-Györgyi about a forty-four-year-old friend diagnosed with cancer of the prostate and treated with surgery and radiation.[16] Unfortunately, the cancer spread to the pelvic bone and the friend was told he had only about a year to live. Luckily, Dr. Stone was one of the first researchers to appreciate that vitamin C may be beneficial in cancer, both for prevention and for treatment.[17] His letter provides an anecdotal account of a patient's use of oral doses of vitamin C in cancer:

Since he began taking 80 grams a day in 1979, his well-being has been excellent. He says he feels great most of the time, has also been able to continue working every day, and lives a fairly normal life [in] the years since November 1978 when orthodox medicine said he would be dead.

Visually, he looks more like an athlete than a terminal cancer patient. . . . In the last few weeks, he has been able to improve his well-being by increasing his ascorbate intake to 130 to 150 grams per day! He has been taking oral doses every hour of 5 to 10 grams of a mixture of nine parts sodium ascorbate plus one part ascorbic acid dissolved in water. [Doses at these short intervals would produce a sustained high level of ascorbate in the tissues as well as in the blood (dynamic flow).] These doses are well tolerated and within bowel tolerance and he has had no trouble from diarrhea, except just lately when he had to reduce the 150 grams a day to 130 grams.

I believe his case is a classic and a good demonstration that if sufficient ascorbate is given to fully counteract all the incident stresses, then the cancer can be controlled. If given early enough in this disease, then cancer may no longer be a problem. Up to now, we just haven't realized how big these daily controlling doses have to be.

Dr. Stone understood that high doses of vitamin C need to be given at short intervals. The massive doses described are typical of those reported to be successful in treating illness.[18] He describes how the man's doctor ran some ascorbate tests on the patient's blood and came up with the highest blood levels he had ever seen—35 mg percent! The so-called normal population averages 1 mg percent or less and the kidney threshold is 1.4 mg percent. Dr. Stone stated that "I would like to see a crash ascorbate program started on terminal cancer patients using doses in the ranges found to keep his cancer under control. Since these 'terminals' have been abandoned by orthodox medicine, they have nothing to lose but their ill health."

The blood level that Dr. Stone describes for the kidney threshold (1.4 mg percent) corresponds to a blood level of about 80 µM/L, which has since been confirmed by results from the National Institutes of Health.[19] This is a minimum baseline level that the body retains to prevent acute scurvy.[20] The level of 35 mg percent corresponds to an amount twenty-five times greater (1,980 µM/L), far larger than the maximum values normally reported in healthy people. Dr. Stone's initial report of benefit to a cancer patient from oral doses of ascorbate at 80–150 grams a day is striking; his finding of such high measured blood levels of ascorbate from an oral dose is astounding.

In May 1984, Dr. Stone was to attend a meeting of the Orthomolecu-lar Medical Society and the Academy of Orthomolecular Psychiatry in Los Angeles, where he was to receive the Linus Pauling Award in honor of his achievements. Unfortunately, he died the night before the meeting, most likely from a heart attack. In his immensely productive 77-year lifetime, Irwin Stone, building on the work of Dr. Szent-Györgyi, constructed the theoretical and practical foundations of orthomolecular medicine. As is often the case, such pioneers are overlooked, and Dr. Stone died only hours before he was to gain a little of the recognition he deserved.

Frederick R. Klenner

Frederick R. Klenner, M.D. (1907–1984), was born in Pennsylvania, and received his undergraduate and Masters degrees in biology from St. Vin-cent and St. Francis Colleges. He earned his doctorate in medicine from Duke University in 1936. Three years later, following his hospital residen-cy, he entered private practice in Reidsville, North Carolina, where he lived for the rest of his life.

In 1946, Dr. Klenner delivered the Fultz quadruplets, the first quadru-plets to survive in the southern states. Before the advent of fertility drugs, the birth was unusual enough for Universal Pictures to send a film crew. Annie Penn Hospital, where they were born, had few modern facilities and was ill equipped for multiple births. In place of an incubator, Dr. Klenner used cotton gauze blankets and placed the children together to share body heat. Notably, they were born under a high vitamin C regimen, which might have contributed to their survival. The mother, Anne Marie, was a deaf mute from a tenant farm without running water and already had six children.

Following the tradition of early medical scientists, Dr. Klenner often experimented on himself with large doses of vitamin C. His particular spe-cialty was diseases of the chest, which led to his interest in vitamin C for viruses. By 1948, he had published his first paper on vitamin C and the treatment of viral disease. Just a year later, he presented a paper to the American Medical Association detailing the complete cure of sixty polio patients using intravenous sodium ascorbate and oral supplementation.

Dr. Klenner's doses of ascorbate were massive, up to 300 grams (over half a pound) per day. He published a series of articles covering the use of vitamin C in treating more than thirty diseases. According to Dr. Klenner, the effects of vitamin C were so universal and striking that, whatever the disease, the doctor's first response should be to give vitamin C. Dr. Klenner spent forty years using vitamin C to treat numerous serious illnesses, including pneumonia, herpes, mononucleosis, hepatitis, multiple sclerosis, childhood illnesses, fevers, and encephalitis. Patients and orthodox physicians are often amazed when they learn that Dr. Klenner employed over 1,000 mg of vitamin C per kilogram body weight per day.

One can only speculate on how much suffering might have been avoided if doctors in the 1950s had listened to him. However, Dr. Klenner did inspire Linus Pauling and Irwin Stone to expand the research on the wider benefits of vitamin C.

Dr. Klenner's Legacy

Dr. Klenner's medical papers, some dating from the 1940s, provide an outstanding contribution to our understanding of vitamin C as a medicine.[21] Even now, the antibiotic and antiviral effects of massive doses of vitamin C are largely unappreciated and unexplored by the health professions. Much of our knowledge in this area originated with Dr. Klenner, whose life was as eventful as a Hollywood melodrama. Dr. Klenner's work is astounding and its nature can be appreciated by the response of Tom Levy, M.D., in his book *Vitamin C, Infectious Diseases, and Toxins: Curing the Incurable*:

> When I first came across Klenner's work on polio patients, I was absolutely amazed and even a bit overwhelmed at what I read. . . . To know that polio had been easily cured and so many babies, children, and some adults still continued to die or survive to be permanently crippled by this virus was extremely difficult to accept. . . . Even more incredibly, Klenner briefly presented a summarization of his work on polio at the Annual Session of the American Medical Association on June 10, 1949 in Atlantic City, New Jersey: "It might be interesting to learn how poliomyelitis was treated in Reidsville, N.C., during the 1948 epidemic. In the past seven years, virus infections have been treated and cured in a period of seventy-two hours by the employment of massive frequent injections of ascorbic acid, or vitamin C. I believe that if vitamin C in these massive doses—6,000 to 20,000 mg in a 24-hour period—is given to these patients with

poliomyelitis none will be paralyzed and there will be no further maiming or epidemics of poliomyelitis."[22]

Dr. Klenner described a cure for what was then arguably the infectious disease most feared by parents in the industrialized world. There was, curiously, no response from the doctors attending the association meeting. While the medical community ignored him, his work did receive some recognition from the local media. *Greensboro Daily News* reporter Flontina Miller wrote:

> Dr. Klenner remembers using [ascorbate] for a man who was lying near death from severe virus pneumonia, but refused to be hospitalized. "I went to his house and gave him one big shot with five grams or 5,000 milligrams of vitamin C," he recalled. "When I went back later in the day, his temperature was down three degrees and he was sitting on the edge of the bed eating. I gave him another shot of C, 5,000 milligrams, and kept up that dosage for three days, four times a day. And he was well. I said then, well, my gosh! This is doing something."[23]

Similar effects of vitamin C's action in acute infections have been repeatedly reported. For example, the Australian doctor Archie Kalokerinos later made several independent observations replicating Dr. Klenner's results.[24]

"We've used massive doses of vitamins on over 10,000 people over a period of thirty years," said Dr. Klenner, "and we've never seen any ill effects from them. The only effects we've seen have been beneficial." Dr. Klenner's immensely valuable work is his legacy. Linus Pauling said that Dr. Klenner's early papers "provide much information about the use of large doses of vitamin C in preventing and treating many diseases. These papers are still important."[25] Dr. Klenner is justly remembered as the doctor who was the first to boldly assert that "ascorbic acid is the safest and most valuable substance available to the physician" and that patients should be given "large doses of vitamin C in all pathological conditions while the physician ponders the diagnosis."

The media have been obsessively interested in the scandal that rocked Dr. Klenner's family following the doctor's death from heart disease in 1984. Fred Klenner, Jr., known as Fritz, was implicated in the murders of at least five people and died by his own hand in 1985. The tragedy was the subject of a best-selling 1988 book (in which Dr. Klenner is mentioned over fifty times) and a 1994 made-for-TV movie. It is instructive to note that the news media reported on the son's crimes far more than it reported on the father's cures.

Dr. Klenner's work inspired later orthomolecular physicians such as Robert F. Cathcart III, who went on to deliver massive doses of vitamin C to thousands of his patients. Whether overshadowed by scandal or stubbornly ignored by the medical profession, high-dose ascorbate therapy is here to stay. "I have used Dr. Klenner's methods on hundreds of patients," said Lendon Smith, M.D. "He is right."

Lendon H. Smith

If Dr. Klenner was one of the most innovative physicians, Lendon H. Smith, M.D. (1921–2001), was among the most courageous. Dr. Smith was one of the first doctors to unambiguously support high-dose vitamin regimens for children. Such a position did not endear him to fellow members of the American Academy of Pediatrics, so Dr. Smith took orthomolecular therapy directly to the people by way of his newsletter (*The Facts*) and his many popular books, articles, videos, and television appearances (he appeared on *The Tonight Show* sixty-two times and even won an Emmy award).

The man who would become nationally known as "The Children's Doctor" received his M.D. in 1946 from the University of Oregon Medical School. He served in the U.S. Army Medical Corps from 1947 to 1949, then completed pediatric residencies at St. Louis Children's Hospital and Portland's Doernbecker Memorial Hospital. In 1955, Dr. Smith became Clinical Professor of Pediatrics at the University of Oregon Medical Hospital. He would practice pediatrics for thirty-five years before retiring in 1987 to lecture, write, and continue to help make *megavitamin* a household word.

It took over twenty years of medical practice before Dr. Smith first began to use megavitamin therapy. A patient "wanted me to give her a vitamin shot," he writes of an alcoholic woman from 1973. "I had never done such a useless thing in my professional life, and I was a little embarrassed to think that she considered me to be the kind of doctor who would do that sort of thing."[26] "That sort of thing" consisted of an intramuscular injection of B-complex vitamins, which proved successful enough that "she walked past three bars and didn't have to go in." That was the beginning of his conversion from conventional pediatrician to orthomolecular spokesperson.

His first book, *The Children's Doctor*, published in 1969, contains only three mentions of vitamins, and two are negative. However, as he learned about nutritional prevention and megavitamin therapy, he began to discuss it. In his 1979 book, *Feed Your Kids Right*, Dr. Smith recommends up to 10,000 mg of vitamin C during illness. By 1981, in *Foods for Healthy Kids*, he recommends vitamin C to bowel tolerance levels (the maximum tolerated oral dose of vitamin C). But even his relatively mild statements, such as "eat no sugar" and "stress increases the need for vitamin B and C, calcium, magnesium, and zinc" can be a walk on the wild side for conventional physicians. Furthermore, his recommendations of B-complex and vitamin C injections, self-administered by the patient twice a week for three weeks, were not calculated to avoid controversy.

By 1979, Dr. Smith was a *New York Times* best-selling author, and by 1983, he was advocating four-day water fasts, 1,000-microgram injections of B_{12}, and megavitamins for kids. There were no Recommended Dietary Allowance (RDA)–level vitamin recommendations in his books. He was also an outspoken critic of junk food: two of his trademark phrases were "People tend to eat the food to which they are sensitive" and "If you love something, it is probably bad for you."

Dr. Smith became cautious about routine vaccination: "The best advice I can give to parents is to forgo the shots, but make sure that the children in your care have a superior immune system." His alternative recommendation was for children to have an immune-boosting diet: "This requires a sugarless diet without processed foods (and) an intake of vitamin C of about 1,000 milligrams per day for each year of life, up to 5,000 milligrams at age five."[27] He clearly realized the connection between sugar intake and vitamin C. Dr. Smith proclaimed, "If we continue to eat store-bought food, we will have store-bought teeth."[28]

These are big steps for a pediatrician who, thirty-two years earlier, had written that excess vitamin C was a waste and would not prevent colds. Dr. Smith might have had a quiet life as a pediatrician had he held onto such incorrect, but politically safe, beliefs. Because of his promotion of orthomolecular medicine, he was finally compelled to stop practicing in

1987, under pressure from insurance companies and his state's Board of Medical Examiners. Nonetheless, he continued to speak out in favor of megavitamin therapy.

The popularization of orthomolecular medicine by courageous physicians such as Lendon Smith has enabled the benefits of nutritional therapy to reach families with sick children. Dr. Smith's visibility has done wonders to educate and encourage parents to use vitamins to prevent and cure illness. For this, Lendon Smith ranks alongside Dr. Klenner as one of the true pioneers of nutritional medicine.

Claus Washington Jungeblut

In the 1950s and 1960s, children were vaccinated against polio. Many kids feared the needle and were pleasantly surprised to receive a lump of sugar instead. In time, they would learn the name of their benefactor, Albert Sabin, M.D., the man credited with having saved all from the risk of a lifetime of paralysis. Ironically, this live oral vaccine may have become a leading cause of polio as the incidence of the disease was reduced.[29] The strongest criticism of Sabin's live vaccine originated from another hero in the fight against polio and developer of an early "killed" polio vaccine, Jonas Salk, M.D. In September 1976, the *Washington Post* reported Dr. Salk's assertion that the Sabin live oral virus vaccine had been the "principal if not sole cause" of every reported polio case in the United States since 1961.[30] In 1996, a year after Dr. Salk died, the U.S. Centers for Disease Control (CDC) began to turn away from the live oral vaccine and recommended killed virus injections for the first two rounds of infant polio immunization. By 2000, the CDC stated that "to eliminate the risk for vaccine-associated paralytic poliomyelitis, an all-injected polio virus schedule is recommended for routine childhood vaccination in the United States."[31] Only after two decades did the orthodoxy at last take heed of the Dr. Salk's caution.

Many people know the names of Drs. Salk and Sabin. By contrast, the public and orthodox medicine are yet to pay proper attention to the work of Claus Washington Jungeblut, M.D. (1898–1976). Dr. Jungeblut received his M.D. from the University of Bern in 1921 and then conducted research at the Robert Koch Institute, in Berlin. A bacteriologist for the New York State Department of Health from 1923 until 1927, he taught at Stanford University and then joined the faculty at Columbia University College of

Physicians and Surgeons. Dr. Jungeblut retired in 1962 and he died in 1976 at the age of seventy-eight. For seven decades, he influenced the course of every nutritional medicine practitioner and earned the thanks of patients whose health and lives were saved by ascorbate therapy.

In his day, Dr. Jungeblut was regarded as an important player in polio research. While recent revisionist history of the fight against polio has generally downplayed his contribution, it has sidestepped what was arguably his most important discovery—that vitamin C may prevent and cure polio. Amazingly, Dr. Jungeblut first published this idea in 1935, shortly after vitamin C had been identified and isolated.[32] His research on vitamin C was sweeping and profound, extending well beyond the topic of polio. By 1937, he had shown that vitamin C inactivated both diphtheria and tetanus toxins.[33] Dr. Jungeblut's research suggested that vitamin C could inactivate toxins and protect against viral and bacterial pathogens, including polio, hepatitis, herpes, and staphylococcus.[34] In September 1939, a *Time* magazine article described how Dr. Jungeblut, while studying statistics of a recent polio epidemic in Australia, deduced that low vitamin C status was associated with the disease.[35] The popular and professional media rarely highlight Dr. Jungeblut's work. Even when he and his work are memorialized, there is no mention of vitamin C.

What Happened to Vitamin C as a Therapy for Polio?

Dr. Jungeblut performed experiments that suggested vitamin C was greatly beneficial in monkeys with polio. Dr. Sabin, who was interested in producing a vaccine at that time, failed to replicate Dr. Jungeblut's results. However, Dr. Sabin effectively prevented a positive result by using larger doses of virus and smaller doses of vitamin C; he also gave the vitamin C far less frequently.[36] Decades later, we have the research base to understand how it is possible to gain a negative result using low and infrequent doses of vitamin C. The process of investigating inadequate doses continues in research to this day, resulting in the continued impression that vitamin C is ineffective even against the common cold, never mind polio.[37]

Dr. Jungeblut demonstrated that ascorbic acid inactivates the polio virus. Shortly afterward, scientists found that other viruses were also inactivated, including vaccinia, foot and mouth disease, rabies, bacteriophage, and tobacco mosaic virus. At sufficiently high doses, vitamin C appears to act as a broad-spectrum antiviral agent. When discussion about poliomyelitis turns toward vitamin C as a prophylaxis and treatment, one hears a frequent refrain: "If vitamin C therapy were so good, all doctors would be using it." However, the doses of vitamin C studied by conventional medical researchers have been too small and too infrequent to be effective.[38] Dr. Sabin's poorly conducted experiments convinced experts that vitamin C was ineffective, clearing the way for a polio vaccine[39] and effectively stopping Dr. Jungeblut's research.[40] Our loss has been a sixty-year period in which vitamin C's antiviral effects have been ignored.

William J. McCormick

Charles Darwin had a far easier time with the acceptance of evolution than physicians have had gaining recognition for the therapeutic use of vitamin C. Vitamin C is needed to make collagen and strong connective tissue, and vitamin C supplementation rapidly enhances collagen synthesis.[41] Some fifty years ago, Toronto physician William J. McCormick, M.D. (1880–1968), pioneered the idea that vitamin C deficiency was a cause of diverse conditions, from stretch marks to cardiovascular disease to cancer.

Stretch Marks

Dr. McCormick suggested that stretch marks are a result of vitamin C deficiency, affecting the body's production of collagen. Collagen consists of long protein molecules that act like tiny strings, holding the tissue components together. We can think of connective tissues as biological fiber composites, working in a similar way to fiberglass or carbon fiber materials. In fiberglass, the plastic matrix is given strength by transferring tension to the glass fibers. Similarly, tissues transfer stress to collagen fibers. Tissues in the body are constructed of cells, supported by a matrix of connective tissue. The cells themselves are relatively delicate and have little intrinsic strength. Connective tissue provides the glue that binds your cells together, just as mortar binds bricks. If collagen is abundant and strong, body cells hold together well. Stretch marks, a relatively minor cosmetic affliction, helped develop Dr. McCormick's ideas. As long ago as 1948, he suggested that these disfiguring lesions might be avoided.[42] During pregnancy, the skin can stretch to several times its original length. If the skin of the abdomen and thighs were stronger and more able to repair itself, stretch marks may be lessened or avoided altogether.

Cancer

It is a large, though logical, step to propose that if cells stick together in a tough, fibrous matrix, tumors might have a hard time spreading through them. Dr. McCormick appears to have been the first person to connect scurvy with a predisposition to cancer.[43] His idea was that growth of tumors would be impeded by a strong connective tissue support matrix. Furthermore, cancer cells could be bound to the matrix, or anchored, so that they could not spread. Consistent with this idea, Dr. McCormick was among the first to report that cancer sufferers typically had very low levels of vitamin C.

Dr. McCormick observed that the symptoms of the classic vitamin C deficiency disease, scurvy, closely resemble those of some types of leukemia and other forms cancer. Today, although scurvy is conventionally considered virtually extinct, cancer is all too prevalent. If the signs of cancer and scurvy are similar, could they be the same disease under different names?[44] James Lind, in his famous experiments on scurvy in the eighteenth century, had noted that the symptoms of the disease were similar to the plague. Dr. McCormick thought that there were also similarities to malignant cancer. For example, the collagen matrix surrounding a tumor breaks down, disturbing the tight arrangement of cells and facilitating ease of spread.[45] He also noted an obscure but interesting reference in the 1905 edition of *Nothnagel's Encyclopedia of Practical Medicine,* which described the similarities between acute lymphatic leukemia and scurvy: "The most striking clinical symptoms of this disease are the hemorrhages and their sequelae. . . . Every touch produces hemorrhage, making a condition completely identical with that of scurvy."[46]

Dr. McCormick concluded that the major effort against cancer might usefully be aimed at preventing it from spreading around the body by way of this cellular disruption. He suggested the use of vitamin C, since the disruption depended on weakened connective tissue and other aspects of tissue structure for which ascorbic acid is essential. This simple hypothesis became the foundation for the therapeutic approach of Linus Pauling and Ewan Cameron, M.D., detailed in their 1979 book *Cancer and Vitamin C,* which used large doses of vitamin C to fight cancer. After all, if cancer cells are going to try to metastasize and spread, abundant vitamin C might strengthen the collagen and connective tissues to keep them from doing so.

It turns out that these mechanisms are not primarily involved in vitamin C's anticancer action, but Dr. McCormick's hypothesis led to some exciting experimentation.[47] The current interest in vitamin C as an anticancer agent began with the investigation of these ideas.

Cardiovascular Disease

One of the early signs of scurvy is bleeding from the gums, as vitamin C is needed to maintain tissue strength and fight disease. Dr. McCormick suggested that a similar process occurs in arteries throughout the body: an artery wall that is short of vitamin C might literally bleed into itself. He reviewed the nutritional causes of heart disease and noted that four out of five coronary cases in hospitals showed vitamin C deficiency. Dr. McCormick was suggesting that heart disease was a form of scurvy,[48] and this association of coronary heart disease with gum inflammation is still an area of active research.[49]

Dr. McCormick was not alone in relating vitamin C to heart disease. As early as 1941, other researchers realized that coronary thrombosis patients had low vitamin C levels.[50] In one study, over half of the patients in a general ward also had low vitamin C status. Arterial plaque, the ultimate cause of heart attack, was known to be associated with capillary hemorrhage. This led to the suggestion that heart disease patients should be provided with adequate amounts of vitamin C. Of course, the definition of "adequate vitamin C" has been at the heart of a nutritional controversy ever since. Supplementation with even a moderate quantity of vitamin C may prevent disease and save lives—just 500 mg daily has been reported to lower mortality from all causes, including heart disease.[51]

Other Beneficial Effects

Dr. McCormick proposed vitamin C deficiency as the essential cause of, and supplementation an effective cure for, numerous communicable illnesses. To support his case, he cited mortality tables from as early as 1840 and suggested that death from tuberculosis, diphtheria, scarlet fever, whooping cough, rheumatic fever, and typhoid fever was primarily due to inadequate dietary vitamin C.[52] To suggest that historical disease trends might relate to a shortage of vitamin C intake appears as novel an idea today as it was nearly sixty years ago. Despite this, the major part of the decline in death rates from infectious disease is generally attributed to sanitation, hygiene, and unspecified improvements in nutrition.

Dr. McCormick considered vitamin C to be the pivotal therapeutic nutrient. He suggested that vitamin C could act both as an antioxidant and, occasionally, as an oxidant within the body.[53] Vitamin C's oxidation-reduction effects provide a powerful chemotherapeutic action, especially when given in large, gram-level doses at hourly intervals. Dr. McCormick noted that the effect was more pronounced when ascorbate was injected, which is remarkably close to our viewpoint on ascorbic acid today. He went further, though, suggesting that the action of vitamin C was comparable to that of antibiotics. Moreover, vitamin C had the advantage of avoiding toxic or allergic reactions, which are common with antibiotics. If the acute symptoms of an infectious disease are controlled by massive doses of vitamin C, the dose can be reduced to a maintenance level. Dr. McCormick made an analogy with extinguishing a fire: a small chemical extinguisher may put out a fire in its early stages, but if the fire is established, large high-pressure fire hoses may be needed.

Ever since Linus Pauling began publicizing the value of megadoses of vitamin C in the early 1970s, it has been a cornerstone of medical mythology that vitamin C can cause kidney stones. The accusation is false.[54] Everybody has heard about unicorns and can describe one in detail, yet unicorns are imaginary, without substance or supporting evidence. Just like a vitamin C kidney stone. Writers often neglect the fact that Dr. McCormick was using vitamin C to prevent and cure kidney stones as far back as 1946.[55] He had observed that cloudy urine was associated with low vitamin C intakes. When such subjects were provided with a large gram-level dose of vitamin C, their urine became clear.

Before the relationship between smoking and both lung cancer and heart disease was established, smoking was often considered a benign pastime. Contrary to this, Dr. McCormick estimated that smoking a single cigarette would oxidize up to 25 mg of vitamin C, about the amount found in a good quality organic orange.[56] This was quite a statement in 1954, a time when physicians were endorsing their favorite cigarette in magazines and on television commercials. Dr. McCormick suggested a heavy smoker could not maintain a healthy level of vitamin C from diet alone. Indeed, if this figure was accurate, a pack-a-day adult smoker taking less than 500 mg of vitamin C per day would soon succumb to acute scurvy or other serious disease related to shortage of vitamin C. (Fortunately, some of this oxidized vitamin C can be regenerated by body tissues.) This and similar estimates of vitamin C loss in smokers are now part of our popular culture, although their author has faded from memory.

Dr. McCormick fought vitamin C deficiency wherever his clinical experience found it. He used gram-sized doses to combat what are usually regarded as non-deficiency-related illnesses. This early therapy set the stage for today's use of therapeutic doses of 100 grams a day to fight cancer and viral disease. For an idea with such potential benefit, the spread of this knowledge has been exceptionally slow. Without Dr. McCormick's published work, it might never have spread at all.

Linus Pauling

Linus Pauling, Ph.D., (1901–1994) was arguably the most highly qualified, and certainly the best known, critic of the vitamin C–deficient medical system. Dr. Pauling still generates extreme reactions, described in terms ranging from "genius" to "quack." His two unshared Nobel Prizes (he is the only person in history with that distinction) are no protection against his opponents, who condemn his approach to the use of vitamins. Dr. Pauling's ideas are considered controversial because he dared to present, directly to the public, his insightful interpretation of the scientific literature suggesting that high doses of vitamins can cure diseases. He also reassessed many "vitamins are useless" studies, explaining how researchers had misinterpreted their own data or presented biased opinions, thus showing that vitamin therapy did indeed have statistically significant value.

Dr. Pauling's contribution is crucial to the story of vitamin C. Strangely, his starting point was to claim that vitamin C could prevent and treat the common cold. From here, he went on to argue that all infectious diseases could be helped with the vitamin: high-dose vitamin C could be considered analogous to an antibiotic, but it would work on viruses as well as bacteria, and would strengthen the immune system. Going further, he claimed that all disease could be helped by vitamin C. Atherosclerosis, the underlying cause of heart disease and stroke, he explained, was caused by vitamin C deficiency. Finally, Dr. Pauling stated that cancer patients would live far longer, or might even be cured, with a sufficient intake of vitamin C.

Since such claims are far beyond the day-to-day experience of most physicians, it is hardly surprising that the medical profession thought Dr. Pauling had lost his way. These ideas, however, did not begin with him— several independent scientists and physicians had witnessed the remarkable properties of vitamin C. Dr. Pauling's contribution was to place these observations within an evolutionary context and to stake his scientific reputation on vitamin C.

The Case for High Vitamin Doses

Dr. Pauling considered how animals use vitamin C. Animals that synthesize vitamin C make relatively large amounts; for example, rats reportedly make 70 mg per kilogram of body weight each day. If a rat is stressed, the amount of ascorbate it produces increases, to about 215 mg per day.[57] However, this is insufficient to maintain vitamin C levels in sick animals, and as blood levels fall, urinary excretion increases by a factor of ten.[58] An injection of vitamin C—a dose roughly equivalent to about 5 grams (5,000 mg) in a human—restores the plasma ascorbate level, blood pressure, and capillary perfusion to normal, while inhibiting bacterial growth. Other animals also increase their vitamin C production when stressed.[59] A plausible explanation is that sick animals increase both the manufacture of vitamin C and its excretion. The rate of ascorbic acid production in the rat is equivalent to a dose of between 5 grams and 15 grams per day, given intravenously, to a 154-pound (70 kg) adult human. Similar rates of production are found in goats and other animals. Domesticated cats and dogs produce somewhat less (human equivalent, 2.5 grams). By way of comparison, the RDA in the United States is less than 0.1 gram per day, between 50 and 150 times lower. Furthermore, oral vitamin C is only partly absorbed.

A direct comparison between the amounts required by animals and humans could be misleading. Humans might have evolved to need less, for example. Dr. Pauling used an evolutionary argument and estimated that the amount of vitamin C in 110 raw plant foods, supplying 2,500 calories, is at least thirty-five times the RDA. However, there is little data on the diet of early man or other mammals. While it is likely that plants 40 million years ago had similar levels of vitamin C to those we find today, we do not have direct measurements. Our ancestors may have been largely vegetarian, though we cannot be certain about this.

Animals that do not synthesize vitamin C may eat a vegetarian diet, providing a high level of the vitamin. However, we cannot be sure that this is always the case, as we do not have a complete list of such animals. We do know that primates, other than humans, consume large amounts of vitamin C in their mainly vegetarian diet. A pet or laboratory monkey is assumed to need the equivalent of 1 gram of vitamin C per day, far more than governments recommend for humans. A wild gorilla eats vegetation containing about 4.5 grams of vitamin C each day. Despite these reservations, Dr. Pauling assumed a diet similar to that of the great apes and calculated the early human intake of vitamin C as somewhere between 2.3 grams and 9.5 grams per day.[60] He suggested that unless it could be shown that our biochemistry is substantially different from our nearest animal relatives, humans should probably be consuming gram-level doses of vitamin C, every day.

Dr. Pauling became convinced that there was a scientific case for high doses of vitamin after listening to Dr. Irwin Stone's ideas. According to Dr. Stone, people need vitamin C in large quantities to deal adequately with infection and stress. Drs. Stone and Pauling thought vitamin C, as ascorbic acid, is required in the diet because of an identifiable genetic mutation, which could be classed as an inborn error of metabolism.

"The Vitamin C Man"

A small number of nutritionists do not regard ascorbic acid to be vitamin C, but instead talk of a "vitamin C complex." There is no supporting evidence for this approach, as L-ascorbic acid given alone will both prevent and cure scurvy. The finding of explanations in the simplest possible form is a central part of the scientific method. Occam's razor, from William of Ockham in the fourteenth century, is applied to both philosophy and science: Put simply, it states that all things being equal, the simplest explanation is preferred. Suggestions that vitamin C is some ill-defined mixture of natural substances is unscientific, although it may be profitable to the commercial organizations concerned.

People consuming the low RDA levels of vitamin C may be considered deficient. Authorities who claim that we only need such small amounts should be required to provide solid data to show that low doses are optimal. Unless such data is produced, official advice may be subjecting millions of people to unnecessary ill health.[61] There is a bias at the heart of conventional nutritional advice. The original hypothesis for a vitamin was that it was a substance required in small amounts to maintain good health. This definition has carried through into modern medicine and it has come to be regarded as fact. People have forgotten that the idea that vitamins were needed in only small amounts was a relative measure, comparing the amount of vitamins to the proportion of fat, protein, and carbohydrate in typical foods. We are now in the unfortunate position where the idea has become a medical dogma.

For decades, it was assumed (without any supporting evidence) that acute scurvy was the only vitamin C deficiency disease. The idea that long-term deficiency could result in chronic illnesses, such as cataracts, heart disease, or arthritis, was largely ignored because there was no "proof" for this suggestion. Dr. Pauling argued for an increased requirement for vitamin C, using comparative biochemistry and evolutionary data. He believed that people had enough vitamin C in the diet to prevent them dying or becoming sick from acute scurvy, but insufficient to prevent disease in the longer term.

Linus Pauling brought the claims for high-doses of vitamin C to the public and named a new form of nutritional therapy—orthomolecular medicine. After a stellar career as one of the greatest scientists ever, he was happy to be known as "the vitamin C man."

These and other scientists and medical doctors have fought over the decades to make a case for high doses of vitamin C to fight disease. While they remained marginalized by the conventional medical community, their courageous struggle has brought the many benefits of vitamin C to the attention to a wider public and, in the process, saved many from needless suffering.

CHAPTER 3

Taking Vitamin C

"What makes ascorbate truly unique is that very large amounts can act as a non-rate-limited antioxidant free radical scavenger."
—ROBERT F. CATHCART III

Many nutritionists refer to the Recommended Dietary Allowance (RDA) by an alternative name—"ridiculous dietary allowance."[1] The rationale behind the official RDA for vitamin C is the prevention of acute scurvy, but it ignores the mounting evidence that higher doses provide more optimal health. A general assumption used in deriving the RDA was that people's individual requirements do not vary greatly. Thus, the RDA does not cover the needs of the sick, the elderly, or others who may need far greater amounts. Having sufficient vitamin C to prevent acute scurvy means that collagen synthesis is sufficient to provide the body with a minimal structural integrity. However, this level of intake, which prevents sickness and death in the short term, has little relevance to the question of the optimal intake for disease prevention. People consuming RDA levels may be endangering their well-being, and even their lives, because of a chronically deficient intake of vitamin C.

The core dispute that has made vitamin C so controversial over the years concerns the optimal intake. Scientists have been unsure how much a person needs for the greatest health benefits. Fortunately, recent research has thrown light on this dark corner of nutrition. One confounding factor is that each person is biologically unique. It may be impossible to specify a single intake to cover the needs of a large population. A second factor is the age and state of health of the individual. Some healthy people might tolerate only a couple of grams (2,000 mg) of vitamin C but,

41

when physiologically stressed, that tolerance might increase 50-fold, or even 100-fold.

Errors in Determining the RDA

A few milligrams a day of vitamin C will prevent acute scurvy. In the short term, a person consuming this small amount will not become ill or die through scurvy. This fact forms the basis of the argument that humans need only a few milligrams a day for good health. Since prevention of the deficiency disease requires only micronutrient amounts of ascorbate, it was classified as vitamin C.

At the time, there was no convincing evidence to show that doses higher than milligram levels were needed. In the 1990s, Mark Levine, M.D., at the U.S. National Institutes of Health (NIH) showed that a healthy adult taking less than about 200 mg of vitamin C each day would have a deficient blood level. By giving varied doses to medical student volunteers, Dr. Levine was able to show that the body attempts to maintain a minimum level in the blood (the body retains 60–80 µM/L in blood plasma). If the intake falls below this level, molecular pumps in the kidney reabsorb vitamin C to prevent loss in urine. These pumps are highly effective: it takes between one and six weeks without vitamin C to reduce the blood concentration to half its original value. These pumps are essential to prevent acute scurvy in times of vitamin C shortage.

The NIH stated that these levels of retention in the blood suggest a required intake of about 200 mg of vitamin C per day. As well as blood plasma levels, Dr. Levine also measured the vitamin C in white blood cells. These cells have molecular pumps in their outer membranes, which are similar to those in the kidney. A white blood cell can accumulate a higher level of vitamin C than the surrounding plasma by actively absorbing the molecule. Dr. Levine found that white blood cells were less sensitive than plasma to intakes of vitamin C. Indeed, compared to plasma, white blood cells need only about half the vitamin C intake (100 mg) to reach their anti-scurvy retention level. This level was used for the RDA and, superficially at least, it appeared to be a rational basis for the new value. However, we need to examine the issue further.

The body has two lines of defense against scurvy. First, the kidney pumps retain a minimum level of vitamin C in the body. However, some tissues, such as brain, adrenal glands, and white blood cells, are more sensitive to vitamin C loss. These cells, which have a specific and essential requirement for vitamin C, have special vitamin C pumps that allow them to preserve higher levels than other tissues. In times of shortage, these tissues maintain their high internal concentrations, whereas blood plasma and less sensitive tissues become deficient. As a person loses vitamin C, most of their body tissues become deficient, though the critical cells and tissues that need it most are protected. Only late in the illness will these essential tissues become greatly deficient. By this time, the person will be suffering severe symptoms and will be close to death.

The use of specialized tissues such as white blood cells for determining the RDA is a gross error.[2] In a person consuming these recommended low intakes of vitamin C per day, the majority of tissues may be deficient. Indeed, the plasma level could often fall below the threshold levels sustained by the kidneys. Had Dr. Levine used red instead of white blood cells, the recommendations would have been completely different. Red blood cells are more numerous than white cells and are not specialized in their use of vitamin C. Red blood cells do not become "saturated" with vitamin C at daily intakes of 100 mg, but would continue to absorb the vitamin at much higher intake levels. Red blood cells are affected by scurvy sooner than white cells. They provide a more appropriate estimate for the RDA, as they are similar to the majority of the body's tissues. A dietary allowance based on red blood cells would prevent earlier signs of scurvy. If scientists need an easily obtainable tissue to determine the optimal human intake, red blood cells would be more suitable than white cells.

Risk-Averse Experts

For over fifty years, governments have felt it necessary to provide nutritional guidance to their populations. Unfortunately, they possessed insufficient data to make a considered argument for many of the nutrients, especially vitamin C. Governments are not particularly good at admitting ignorance and typically select their committees from scientists who support the status quo. Furthermore, scientists on such committees may feel that they are required to be conservative. Rather than making an objective assessment of potential health benefits, committee members may think they are steering on the side of safety by recommending an intake that is as low as possible without an individual being at risk of acute scurvy.

By recommending a minimal dose, governments risk specifying a grossly inadequate intake. Healthy people who consume just a few milligrams a day will not die or suffer the acute effects of scurvy. At intakes of 40–60 mg per day, specialized tissues such as brain and white blood cells may maintain high internal levels. Thus, government scientists in the United Kingdom, being suitably conservative, set the Dietary Reference Intake (DRI) for adults at 40 mg per day.[3] Their aim was presumably to use the precautionary principle in order to avoid people being poisoned by higher doses. (There is no evidence for such effects from vitamin C, however.) The U.S. Food and Nutrition Board also based their RDA on the amount needed to prevent acute scurvy. The RDAs exclude people with special needs, which may be anyone who is elderly, ill, or stressed. However, they are applied generally to the whole population.

The official aim of the RDA or DRI is to recommend the intake with minimum risk of inadequacy and toxicity. Since there is remarkably little danger from high doses of vitamin C, we might expect the data for the recommended intake to be strongly influenced by potential beneficial effects. However, in the bizarre world of bureaucratic logic, beneficial effects are often excluded from the analysis of requirements. Instead of a well-founded approach based on the available data, the recommendations are essentially based on risk analysis. Risk analysis is useful for the dangers of toxic substances in the environment, but is inadequate when considering a substance essential to life. Such recommendations are biased against higher doses, because theoretically they could always be dangerous in some unspecified way.

Science and common sense suggests that a single RDA for vitamin C, or any other vitamin, is unlikely to be adequate for the population. Humans are biologically diverse and such biodiversity implies some people would need far more than the recommended doses. This variation in requirements can also occur within a single individual, as needs may change with illness or age.

Government values do not consider long-term effects of deprivation, although even intakes several times the RDA might be associated with chronic disease. For example, atherosclerosis and heart disease could be a result of chronic subclinical scurvy.[4] Governments have no evidence that chronic disease is not a result of their low recommendations. Investigating the long-term effects of vitamin C deprivation is difficult and expensive. Without this evidence, the recommendations rely on the opinions of experts. Yet, if subclinical scurvy causes chronic disease, we will all suffer the consequences of doses that are too low. If governments would admit the level of uncertainty in their recommendations, people would at least be able to reach their own conclusions.

Factors Affecting Vitamin C Absorption

Dr. Levine hoped to solve the problem of vitamin C requirements using biochemistry. He suggested that vitamin C requirements could be found by experiment.[5] His idea was to estimate the optimal intake by finding out how much of a dose is absorbed or excreted—someone who is taking in too much vitamin C might not absorb it or might excrete it rapidly.

At that time, scientists knew little about how doses of vitamin C traveled around the body. There was some information for healthy, young adults, in whom vitamin C is actively absorbed from the intestine.[6] Almost all of a low dose, below about 60 mg, is absorbed.[7] The absolute amount absorbed increases with dose, but only slowly: up to 80–90 percent of a single 180-mg dose is absorbed, reducing to 75 percent at 1 gram, 50 percent at 1.5 grams, 26 percent at 6 grams, and 16 percent at 12 grams.[8] Only 2 grams of a single 12-gram dose would be absorbed, providing a limit to the intake possible from a single dose. Conversely, only small amounts of low doses are excreted unchanged. As the dose increases, more vitamin C is excreted because the pumps in the kidney are limited in the amount that they can retain.

The NIH proposed an RDA of 200 mg of vitamin C per day for healthy young men. A little later, Dr. Levine obtained similar results for healthy young women. In a series of influential papers, he described the absorption, blood levels, and excretion of vitamin C.[9] These papers form the core evidence used for current government recommendations. The NIH suggested that the body was "saturated" at an intake of 200 mg per day. According to this notion, increasing the dose would not sustain blood levels at a higher value than 60–70 µM/L and the majority of larger doses is not absorbed from the gut. This is clearly an error, as sustained blood levels of at least three times this claimed maximum concentration are achievable with repeated oral doses.

As mentioned previously, vitamin C is not confined to the blood plasma, but is selectively pumped into a number of specialized tissues, including the brain, white blood cells, and the adrenal glands.[10] The cells and

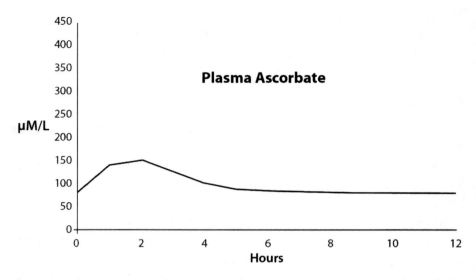

Dose-response curve for blood plasma concentration following a 1,250-mg
dose of vitamin C in a depleted subject.

organs that are protected in this way are essential to survival and have
higher than normal requirements for vitamin C and its antioxidant protection. White blood cells, for example, have specific requirements for vitamin C in fighting infection. These white cells have a short lifespan and
their death is controlled by levels of antioxidants.[11] The pumps in these
tissues ensure that in times of shortage, the vitamin C levels remain high.

At vitamin C intakes below about 100–200 mg per day, the specialized
tissues are protected from scurvy by accumulating high levels relative to
normal tissues. In recommending 200 mg per day, Dr. Levine added that
doses above 400 mg provide no additional benefit. At this suggested
intake, most of the tissues in the body are in a state of depletion. Moreover, intakes of at least 18 grams of vitamin C per day are required to provide the maximum sustained blood levels.[12]

Molecular Pumps and Vitamin C

Vitamin C, or ascorbic acid, is a simple organic molecule similar to glucose. The glucose molecule constitutes a high proportion of the normal
diet, typically many hundreds of grams each day. Notably, the abundant
glucose competes with vitamin C, further limiting ascorbate's benefits.

When glucose (blood sugar) is high, less vitamin C is transported into cells,[13] which may explain why many people do not report positive effects of vitamin C supplementation with the common cold and other illnesses.[14] "Take more vitamin C and eat less sugar and carbohydrates" might be a new adage to replace the basic wisdom of the old one: "Starve a cold, lest you feed a fever." Many high-dose vitamin C tablets or drinks that are laden with sugar in essence provide the antidote with the drug.

The specialized cells in the body that concentrate vitamin C have several types of molecular pump in the cell membrane to transport vitamin C. One type is called GLUT (glucose transporter) and pumps oxidized vitamin C into cells. Oxidized vitamin C (dehydroascorbate) has a similar molecular shape to glucose, hence GLUT pumps can transport either molecule. This pumping is competitive, which means that if there is a lot of glucose, then it will be pumped in preference to oxidized vitamin C.

Two other pumps transport vitamin C into tissues that have high need, including tissues in the intestines, kidney, liver, brain, eye, and other organs.[15] While the pumps have a limited capacity for transporting vitamin C, the cells can become full at relatively low levels in the surrounding fluid. At higher plasma concentrations, the cells continue to accumulate ascorbate, but the rate is low. The possession of ascorbate pumps provides an indication that a cell is particularly sensitive to depletion of the vitamin.

The hormone insulin is able to move GLUT transporters from the interior of a cell to its surface, where more glucose can be transferred.[16] Diabetics, who lack insulin, are unable to manage this increased absorption and sugar accumulates in their blood. One explanation for the long-term symptoms of diabetes is that the person's cells are chronically short of vitamin C. Hormones such as insulin could also affect the body's ability to absorb vitamin C.

We have already described the massive increase in absorption of ascorbate from the gut during stress and illness. Unfortunately, this response has not been investigated and the underlying control mechanisms are unknown.

Dynamic Flow

A single, large dose of vitamin C produces a brief response in the body. Gram-level doses produce a response above the background level (~70 µM/L) and this is rapidly excreted in urine. High concentrations in blood plasma are excreted with a half-life of about thirty minutes. *However, when the dose is repeated, blood plasma levels can increase*. A second dose adds to the blood levels before the previous dose is excreted. Separating doses by less than 3–4 hours can increase the levels to a plateau of about 250 µM/L in a previously deficient subject.

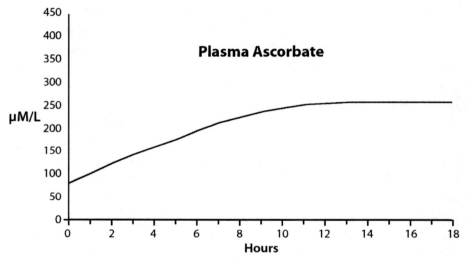

Repeated gram-level doses of vitamin C at hourly intervals produce a steady state in a depleted individual; a sustained maximum level requires an intake of about 20 grams per day.

As a simple analogy, consider a water barrel with a hole part way up the side. Left for a short period without filling, the barrel will settle down to a water level just below the hole (the baseline level). An attempt to fill the barrel with a bucket will only partly succeed. A single bucketful will raise the water level slightly, but it will soon escape through the hole. This is what happens when single doses of vitamin C are given once a day—the blood level is briefly increased, but soon falls back to the baseline. Dynamic flow is equivalent to filling the barrel from a continuously flowing tap. By increasing the flow, leakage from the hole can be overcome and the water level in the barrel can be increased indefinitely.

In dynamic flow, vitamin C is abundant in blood plasma and diffuses slowly into other body compartments. A typical adult human has a blood volume of about five liters. Cells take up somewhat less than half of this volume, with plasma making up the remaining fluid. Red cells are the predominant cell type and slowly absorb vitamin C by diffusion from the plasma. Given time, the concentrations in the plasma and the red blood cells will reach equilibrium. At this point, the blood concentration will have increased to the dynamic flow plateau level or above.

Blood makes up only a small fraction of the tissue volume. In a typical 150-pound (70 kg) human body, about 7 percent of the total volume is blood. High plasma ascorbate levels can diffuse slowly into other tissue compartments. Given time, the body will reach equilibrium, with the tissue levels being equal to or above the mean plasma concentration. When this occurs, the total amount of vitamin C in the body is much greater than that of a person who is not taking regular doses.

If a person who has been in dynamic flow for a considerable period stops taking vitamin C, blood levels remain high until the kidneys excrete the vitamin C. As a result, the vitamin C concentration in the large tissue volume is at a higher level than in the blood plasma, so vitamin C diffuses from the tissues into the blood. Such flow from the tissues sustains the plasma concentration for some time. Moreover, people in dynamic flow who become ill with a common cold or similar infection have a large advantage. Their blood levels are maintained by the frequent oral doses, and at times of high demand, the reserves in their tissues will prevent the blood plasma from being depleted.

The Short Half-Life of Vitamin C

Vitamin C's short plasma half-life means that a large oral dose will raise blood levels for only a few hours. For the rest of the day, the level in blood plasma drops back to the background level of 70 µM/L. For decades, investigations into the properties of vitamin C have been flawed. Many scientists considered a gram-level dose to be large and this idea confuses nutrition and pharmacology. Nutritional intakes are required to maintain optimal health, while pharmacological intakes involve the use of vitamin C as a medicine to treat illness. Nutritional doses are typically considered to be up to about 10 grams per day, whereas 10 grams would be only a small pharmacological dose. For example, Robert F. Cathcart III, M.D., and others have used 40 grams, 60 grams, or even 200 grams a day in divided doses to treat a wide variety of illnesses with apparently great suc-

cess.[17] Many studies on vitamin C and the common cold confuse prevention and treatment, and often doses below 1 gram are studied for both.[18]
The dominant error has been to study single daily doses. Healthy individuals who want protection from the common cold or other illnesses by taking vitamin C need to raise their blood levels by taking divided doses or
slow-release formulations.

What is the Optimal Intake?

The optimal intake for a healthy person has not been established. As we've
seen, much of the work underlying the government RDA is flawed and the
recommended intakes of vitamin C are woefully inadequate. Recent developments have demonstrated that the assumptions upon which the RDA
was based are unjustified and unsupportable. There is currently no evidence to support the idea that low doses of vitamin C are optimal. Indeed,
low intakes may be the cause of much of the world's chronic disease.

Recently, because of the NIH experiments into the uptake and excretion of vitamin C, the RDA was revised from 60 mg daily for adults to 90
mg for men and 75 mg for women. Smokers are recommended to take an
extra 35 mg per day, as the toxins produced by inhaling cigarette smoke
increase oxidative stress and smokers tend to have lower blood levels of
vitamin C anyway. However, this recommendation may be a gross under-
estimate, leaving smokers with a false sense of security—recent observations with large intravenous infusions of sodium ascorbate suggest that
smoking can produce a high degree of oxidation, resulting in lowered plasma ascorbate levels.[19]

A person starting to take vitamin C supplements is starting from a level
of relative deficiency. By taking repeated doses, the levels in the tissues and
blood plasma increase and more can be tolerated. Human requirements for
vitamin C appear to be more variable than previously realized. The key
point is that people need more, far more, than previously assumed. Using
the criteria used to set the RDA, and removing the errors, leads to a suggestion that the intake for a healthy adult should be in the range of about
500 mg to 20 grams (20,000 mg), or even more. Some people would
require low doses and would not tolerate higher intakes; others need higher levels, above 10 grams.

*A person wishing to estimate his or her own requirement needs to deter-
mine their bowel tolerance level.* To do this, start with a low dose and

repeat it each hour until unpleasant bowel effects (gas, distension, and loose stools) are observed. This level of intake is your bowel tolerance level and the optimal intake is 50–90 percent of this maximum. Keep in mind that a high carbohydrate intake can interfere with the bowel tolerance test and falsely indicate a lower limit. Vitamin C requirements change with the state of health and need to be re-checked in this way from time to time. Perhaps more importantly, the level that a person can tolerate increases with time, as dynamic flow is maintained.

People vary in their requirements and it is not possible to provide a definitive statement about intakes that applies to all. Furthermore, a person's requirement will vary, increasing with even a slight illness. The minimum intake required to raise a typical adult's blood plasma levels consistently is 2–3 grams (2,000–3,000 mg) per day, in divided doses of about 500 mg. For some, this will be too high and they may need to lower the dose slightly. For many, this intake will be too low to provide resistance to infections and chronic disease.

Forms of Vitamin C

Vitamin C is available in many formulations and there are numerous claims for more effective supplement brands. Often, the claim is that their particular form of vitamin C has improved absorption when taken orally. Most forms of vitamin C are absorbed at comparable rates, although sustained release forms result in delayed absorption.[20] In some cases, manufacturers claim that they have a more "natural" form of the vitamin, suggesting that theirs is the real vitamin C and ascorbic acid is not the genuine vitamin. Such claims are spurious. Vitamin C is defined as L-ascorbic acid, and in general, this is the vitamin C of choice, which is readily available at low cost. However, there are caveats and advantages associated with other forms.

Natural Vitamin C

Natural vitamin C is the same molecule as synthetic L-ascorbic acid.[21] They are chemically identical with no known differences, whether physical, chemical, or biological, so there is no advantage to supplementing with "natural" vitamin C over L-ascorbic acid.[22] As we have explained, occasionally epidemiological papers and clinical trials suggest that vitamin C in food is more effective than the vitamin C in supplements. However, such suggestions are misplaced, as the molecule is identical.[23] Indeed in some foods, such as broccoli, the absorption may be impaired.[24] Despite suggestions that there may be "magic" factors associated with vitamin C in foods, the differences between vitamin C in foods and supplements can be explained more easily as experimental error, such as underestimating the vitamin C in food. Furthermore, absorption of vitamin C from food can occur more slowly than from supplements, thus increasing average blood levels more effectively.

Natural vitamin C is often found in combination with plant pigments called bioflavonoids. Bioflavonoids are often antioxidants and are found in citrus and other fruits and vegetables with a high vitamin C content. There is some evidence that bioflavonoids increase the availability of vitamin C. However, to be effective, this requires a higher intake of bioflavonoids than is commonly found in vitamin C tablets.[25] At low doses, vitamin C is well absorbed, so the benefits of bioflavonoids are unclear.

Mineral Forms

Since pure vitamin C is a weak acid, combining it with minerals, such as sodium, calcium, or magnesium, produces a non-acidic salt. Several forms of mineral ascorbate are common in supplements, with sodium ascorbate and calcium ascorbate being the most frequent. Some people find mineral forms are easier on the stomach, as they are less acidic. People taking massive doses of vitamin C as a mineral ascorbate may also end up consuming large amounts of the mineral. Sodium ascorbate contains 131 mg of sodium and calcium ascorbate has 114 mg of calcium per gram. Consuming many grams of vitamin C in this form may be contraindicated in some conditions, such as kidney disease.

However, there is a more critical restriction to the consumption of massive doses of mineral ascorbate—these forms are less effective. Sick people can often take massive amounts of vitamin C without significant oral discomfort. At a threshold point, close to bowel tolerance, the symptoms of a common cold, for example, often disappear. However, this threshold effect appears to be limited to vitamin C as ascorbic acid and it is not found with mineral ascorbates. Dr. Cathcart was the first to describe this greater response to ascorbic acid over other forms, which has been confirmed by others. This could be because vitamin C contains two available antioxidant electrons, but in mineral forms of ascorbate this number is lower. In sodium ascorbate, the sodium atom replaces one antioxidant electron. Once absorbed, a molecule of sodium ascorbate needs to gain an electron from the body's metabolism in order to function. This effect may be one reason why some people experimenting with massive doses of ascorbate do not achieve the claimed benefits.

Lipid-Soluble C

Another form of vitamin C, ascorbyl palmitate, is a lipid-soluble form of vitamin C. Unlike the proprietary brand of mineral ascorbates, Ester-C™, it is a true ester. A molecule of ascorbyl palmitate is vitamin C combined (esterified) with the fatty acid palmitate. Ascorbyl palmitate is used as a food additive, but is most commonly found as an ingredient of anti-aging cosmetics because of its antioxidant properties and its role in collagen synthesis.[26] When taken orally, ascorbyl palmitate may be largely converted to L-ascorbic acid and palmitate in the liver, and it is unclear if it provides any advantage over L-ascorbic acid.[27] Ascorbyl palmitate is frequently used in cosmetics and topical preparations.

Liposomal C

For healthy people and many with chronic disease, enough vitamin C is provided by dynamic flow levels attained with inexpensive vitamin C. However, some people with diseases such as cancer may not be able to achieve sufficient levels in the blood to combat the illness with normal vitamin C supplements. Intravenous infusion of sodium ascorbate is one option, but a new oral form, liposomal C, also allows greater blood levels to be attained.

A thin membrane surrounds every cell in the body, constructed of two layers of a fat-like substance called phospholipid. Phospholipids have some of the chemical properties of soap: they contain a polar (water-soluble) head and a non-polar (fat-soluble) tail. The head will dissolve in water and the tail in fat, an arrangement that, in soap, helps break up fat deposits during washing. This molecular arrangement means that phospholipids, like soap, can form bubbles when mixed in water.

Liposomes are formed from bubbles of phospholipids, often containing and protecting a liquid content. Commercially produced liposomes may be very small and can be filled with drugs or supplements as an aid to absorption into the body. They provide a method for overcoming the barrier to oral uptake of vitamin C. We have seen that if a person used to low intakes of vitamin C is given a single dose of 12 grams, only about 2 grams will be absorbed. However, if liposomes are filled with concentrated vitamin C, they can theoretically overcome this absorption limit, delivering most of the 12 grams to the body. The result of a large dose of liposomal vitamin C is a gradual increase in blood levels, similar to that obtained with a standard tablet. However, the peak level may be far higher, above 400 µM/L, and the response is sustained. These spectacularly high plasma levels of vitamin C are selectively toxic to cancer cells and liposomes extend the potential of oral doses to combat disease, including cancer.

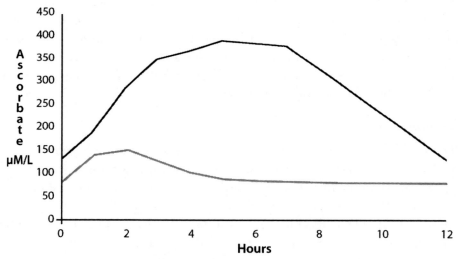

Schematic comparison between the claimed maximal plasma response (to 1,250 mg of vitamin C; *gray line*) to that obtained with an oral dose of 36,000 mg of liposomal ascorbate (*black line*). (Hickey, S., et al. *JNEM* [2008])

Are High Doses of Vitamin C Safe?

The idea that people might want us to accept something false as fact is well-known, as we are bombarded daily with advertising. Much advertising aims at generating such misleading "facts" by frequent repetition. The word *factoid* refers to an item of unreliable information, which has been given credence by repeated exposure. Factoids are "facts" that had no existence before appearing in a magazine or newspaper. At its heart, a factoid is an assumption or speculation. For several decades, an odd medical and media campaign has generated a series of such factoids concerning the safety of vitamin C. Typically, these scare stories are given wide media publicity before they are subjected to scientific scrutiny.

Vitamin C is remarkably safe, which is not surprising considering it is essential to human life and is actively retained in the body. Vitamin C is a simple molecule, used by both animals and plants, often at high concentrations. Organisms have had hundreds of millions of years to evolve mechanisms for prevention of damage by vitamin C. But even allowing for such tolerance, the safety of vitamin C is outstanding. It is unusual in that it can be taken in massive doses, for long periods, without apparent harm.

Vitamins generally have an excellent safety profile—the harmful effects of overdosing are generally overstated. When the science is considered dispassionately, it becomes clear that people are in greater danger of deficiency than overdose. Nevertheless, vitamin intake needs to be considered carefully to ensure optimal nutrition, free from side effects.

The margin of safety for large doses of vitamin C is much greater than that for aspirin, antihistamines, antibiotics, pain medications, muscle relaxants, tranquillizers, sedatives, and diuretics. In other words, vitamin C is far safer than commonly used drugs. However, harmful effects have been wrongly attributed to vitamin C, including hypoglycemia, rebound scurvy, infertility, mutagenesis, and destruction of vitamin B_{12}.[28] We have not found a single validated report of a healthy person dying from a vitamin C overdose in the scientific literature. Not one.

As Safe as Milk

Vitamin C is generally recognized as safe (GRAS). This means that U.S. Food and Drug Administration (FDA) experts consider it can be safely added to food and cosmetics. In the case of food, this is a sensible approach, as without it we would die. Nevertheless, too much vitamin C, like an overdose of water, could be harmful. Taken in excess, water can lower the concentration of sodium in the blood and cause the brain to swell. To put the safety of vitamin C in context, we consider that it might be easier to commit suicide by overdosing on pure water than by eating too much vitamin C.

A review of twenty-three years of U.S. poison control center reports, from 1983 to 2005, indicates that vitamins have been connected with the deaths of only ten people. Indeed, poison control statistics confirm that more Americans die each year from eating soap than from taking vitamins.[29] Even including intentional and accidental misuse, the number of alleged vitamin fatalities is strikingly low, averaging less than one death per year for more than two decades. The American Association of Poison Control Centers (AAPCC), which maintains the U.S. database of information from sixty-one poison control centers, has noted that vitamins are among the most reported substances. The small number of fatalities does not, therefore, reflect a lack of reporting. In sixteen of twenty-three years, the AAPCC reported that there was not a single death due to vitamins.

These statistics specifically include vitamin A, niacin (B_3), pyridoxine (B_6), other B-complex vitamins, vitamins C, D, E, other vitamins such as vitamin K, and multiple vitamins without iron. Minerals, which are chemically and nutritionally different from vitamins, also have an excellent safety record, but not quite as good as vitamins. On the average, one or two fatalities per year are typically attributed to iron poisoning from gross overdosing on supplemental iron. Deaths attributed to other supplemental minerals are very rare. Even iron, although not as safe as vitamins, accounts for fewer deaths than laundry and dishwashing detergents.

ANNUAL DEATHS IN THE U.S. ALLEGED FROM VITAMINS (AAPCC)					
YEAR	ALLEGED DEATHS	YEAR	ALLEGED DEATHS	YEAR	ALLEGED DEATHS
2005	0	1997	0	1989	0
2004	2	1996	0	1988	0
2003	2	1995	0	1987	1
2002	1	1994	0	1986	0
2001	0	1993	1	1985	0
2000	0	1992	0	1984	0
1999	0	1991	2	1983	0
1998	0	1990	1		

The occurrence of even one death should be taken seriously. However, the background details of these reported events are not provided. A human death from an oral overdose of vitamin C in a healthy person does not appear to have been established in the literature. Moreover, a brief consideration of some medical mortality figures places this into context.

Let us consider just those deaths and injuries caused by the effect of aspirin-like drugs (nonsteroidal anti-inflammatory drugs or NSAIDs) on ulcers in older people alone. Note that this is a rather severe restriction in terms of stomach effects and it excludes other age groups. These drugs are often also used for slight headache, muscle strain, and arthritis. Every year, about 41,000 older adults are hospitalized in the U.S. The average stay in the hospital for peptic ulcer in elderly persons is over a week (8.5 days), but about 350,000 unnecessary days in the hospital occurred in 1987 due to NSAIDs.[30] In fact, 3,300 people die every year from these complications.[31] These figures are a challenge to anyone who claims high doses of vitamin C are a health risk. Furthermore, they are only a small fraction of the large number of unnecessary deaths each year from prescription and over-the-counter drugs.

Vitamin C is one of the least toxic substances known. There have been one or two allegations, but nothing confirmed about alleged deaths from vitamin C. The acute safety of a drug is described by the therapeutic index—the toxic dose divided by the therapeutic dose. The Lethal Dose 50 (LD_{50}) is the dose at which 50 percent of the subjects would die. For example, a substance with a therapeutic dose of 1 gram, and an LD_{50} of 2 grams, would have a therapeutic index of 2. Such a low therapeutic index indicates a dangerous drug, with little margin of safety. This kind of drug would be suitable for treatment in only the most severe, life-threatening conditions. The therapeutic index of vitamin C for a 154-pound (70 kg) person taking 1 gram is at least 350, which indicates a high degree of safety. A person who ate a half-pound of vitamin C (227 grams) at a single sitting would probably have trouble with stomach acidity and diarrhea. However, they would be likely to survive.

By way of comparison, the widely available painkiller paracetamol (acetaminophen) has a therapeutic index of about 25. The recommended dose of paracetamol is 1 gram and doses as low as 4 grams can cause serious liver damage.[32] In the U.S., paracetamol overdoses cause about 56,000 emergency room visits and 26,000 hospitalizations each year.[33] Paracetamol causes 458 deaths in these patients each year, many from unintentional overdoses.

At least 16,500 people die each year in the U.S. because of over-the-counter painkillers, and over 100,000 may be hospitalized by their side effects.[34] Medical error is a leading cause of death, reportedly killing at least 100,000 people a year in the U.S.[35] In addition, 12,000 cases of unnecessary surgery, 7,000 errors in giving drugs, 80,000 hospital infections, 106,000 adverse drug reactions, and 20,000 other errors, all lead to avoidable death.[36]

The media give high prominence to vitamin C scare stories, based on little evidence. They often fail to highlight more substantial medical facts, if such information could disturb the status quo.

Potential Side Effects

Does Vitamin C Cause Kidney Stones?

There is no evidence of adverse effects from large amounts of vitamin C.[37] One of the most frequent scare stories is the idea that vitamin C causes kidney stones. Although this originally may have seemed a plausible hypothesis, in practice, high rates of kidney stones are not found in people taking large amounts of vitamin C. Vitamin C has even been proposed and used as a treatment for kidney stones.[38]

The main argument for increased kidney stones relates to those stones formed from calcium oxalate. Unlike some other stone types, these can form in acidic urine, and vitamin C is a weak acid. Calcium oxalate stones make up about three-quarters of all kidney stones. Excess calcium in the urine promotes calcium oxalate stone formation and magnesium inhibits it.[39] High carbohydrate intakes can also increase excretion of calcium.[40] Some researchers have claimed that vitamin C increases the excretion of oxalate in the body slightly, but other studies show no increase in oxalate excretion.[41] It now appears that the higher oxalate levels in some studies are a result of inadequate preservation of samples.

There is a more fundamental problem with these studies of urinary oxalate and calcium. Researchers generated a means of estimating the risk of calcium oxalate formation from the chemical composition of urine.[42] However, this model does not include the effect of vitamin C: the presence of vitamin C in the urine, as expected with high intakes, would lower the risk estimate. The theoretical connection between ascorbate and oxalate stones is based on the Tiselius equation, which relates stone risk to calcium and oxalate and inversely to magnesium. It does not directly include vitamin C. The true situation is that large doses increase ascorbate in urine and this would lower the risk by binding calcium. It is strange indeed that the base argument for vitamin C–associated risk excludes the molecule in question from the analysis. If you include ascorbate at high concentration, the result would be a lower risk of oxalate stones! Thus, many doctors have overestimated the dangers of high-dose vitamin C, which could be protective.

There are additional reasons to suspect that vitamin C may protect against kidney stones. For example, in high doses, it increases urine flow: fast moving rivers deposit little silt. Furthermore, kidney stones appear to form around a nucleus of infection and, since vitamin C at high concentrations is bactericidal, it may remove the focus for stone formation.

Epidemiological evidence suggests vitamin C does not increase kidney stones. A 14-year prospective study of 85,557 women revealed no evidence that vitamin C causes kidney stones.[43] People taking less than 250 milligrams per day and those taking 1.5 grams or more had similar rates of kidney stones. An earlier study of 45,251 men suggested that those taking more than 1.5 grams of vitamin C per day had a *lower* risk of kidney stones.[44]

There are other, less frequent, types of kidney stones, such as those composed of calcium phosphate and struvite (magnesium ammonium phosphate), which can occur in infected urine but which dissolve in acid. Acid urine is produced by vitamin C, which once again may be preventive. Vitamin C is not directly involved in the formation of uric acid stones, found in gout, or cystine stones in children.

Other Side Effects?

There may be interactions with vitamin C in some enzyme deficiencies. In glycogen storage disease (type 1), also known as von Gierke disease, excess glucose is stored in the body as glycogen, from which it can normally be released quickly. This disease sometimes arises from an inherited deficiency of the enzyme glucose-6-phosphate dehydrogenase (G6PD). Some authors claim that this is the most common enzyme deficiency in humans, affecting over 400 million persons worldwide.[45] However, the deficiency disease is actually rare, with an incidence of 1 in 100,000 births in the U.S. Since the gene is sex linked and located on the X chromosome, the deficiency is rare in females. The problem occurs more frequently among people of Mediterranean, African, and Southeast-Asian descent. The incidence in non-Ashkenazi Jews from North Africa may be as high as one case in 5,420 people. The low incidence of clinical enzyme deficiency disease indicates that the condition is rather less common than is normally suggested.

People with G6PD deficiency can suffer glycogen storage disease. Before therapies, such as continuous feeding and the use of cooked cornstarch, most people with this rare condition died young. With improved treatments, more patients are living to adulthood. Even with treatment, people with this disorder have short stature and enlarged livers. Often they suffer from gouty arthritis with kidney stones, increased blood fats, hypertension, acute pancreatitis, osteoporosis, and increased bone fractures.

It has been suggested that a person with this enzyme deficiency who takes high-dose vitamin C supplements could be subject to hemolytic anemia.[46] There is some evidence for this claim in newborn infants, and occasional anecdotal reports in adults.[47] But claims for this side effect have been extrapolated to the extreme and G6PD deficiency causes little risk to healthy people considering high-dose vitamin C.[48]

People suffering from hemochromatosis, or iron overload disease, are claimed to show side effects with high-dose vitamin C. In apparently healthy individuals, vitamin C does not cause excess absorption of iron.[49] However, hereditary hemochromatosis affects about one in 300 people of northern European descent.[50] People with this disease could be adversely affected by long-term ingestion of large doses of vitamin C, although this risk has not been clearly established.[51] There have been one or two case reports of people with hemochromatosis suffering problems with high doses of vitamin C, but considering the large number of supplement takers these reports could simply reflect a chance association. High blood levels of vitamin C in normal, healthy adults and preterm infants, in the presence of iron, do not appear to cause damaging oxidation. Supplementing with vitamin C may prevent such damage, even in iron-overloaded plasma.[52]

These objections to the use of vitamin C have been overstated. Dr. Cathcart, who was one of the most experienced physicians with high-dose vitamin C supplementation, reports direct experience of two patients with hemochromatosis, whom he treated with massive doses of ascorbate without problem. In the thousands of patients he has treated, he has never seen any evidence of a damaging iron-related reaction. His clinical experience indicates that vitamin C increases iron absorption when the body needs it, and he suggests that vitamin C may also increase excretion of iron when there is an excess. He proposes that the vitamin in sufficiently high doses might be an effective treatment for hemochromatosis, which is caused by free radical reactions. The chemistry of vitamin C acting either as an oxidant or as an antioxidant in such conditions is not well understood. While some scientists suggest theoretical problems, others propose beneficial effects. In Dr. Cathcart's words: "This theoretical difficulty concerning C is typical of how the orthodoxy will expand a theory into a fact without any evidence."[53]

The Precautionary Principle

For decades, the medical establishment has accepted the idea that we only need low doses of vitamin C for optimal health. Despite the fact that this idea has little, if any, scientific support, it is now promoted by medical and health organizations worldwide. It is therefore deemed necessary to provide scientific evidence for the alternative hypothesis, that people need high doses. This may be absurd, but it is based on the precautionary principle, which states that a policy should not be implemented unless there is a scientific consensus that it would cause no harm to the public.[54] The burden of "proof" falls on those who advocate the change. A company wanting to release a chemical into the environment, for example, needs to provide solid evidence that it will do no harm. In the case of a potentially harmful new chemical, such an argument is conservative and is based on appropriate caution.

A standard criticism of the precautionary principle is that it only applies to new ideas. In fact, existing procedures may be equally harmful, if not more so. In effect, the precautionary principle states that even if there is no evidence for a side effect, we should still act as though the side effect is possible. Following this principle, you assume the worst case will occur if too large an intake of vitamin C is recommended, and set the guidelines at a minimum level. For radiation, potentially harmful environmental chemicals, and synthetic drugs, this may be conservative. However, when considering nutrients that we cannot live without and are ignorant of how much a person needs for good health, the approach is inappropriate. In the case of vitamin C, the precautionary principle is being misapplied, as there is no evidence that low intakes of vitamin C are less harmful than higher intakes.

When "Side Effects" are Useful

Scientists agree on only one "side effect" for high doses of vitamin C—a single, large dose of vitamin C can be used as a natural laxative. It provides an alternative to drug-based remedies for constipation. At high doses, diarrhea can occur, although the dose needed to produce the effect varies. The level at which diarrhea occurs is called the "bowel tolerance" level and is an indicator of the body's need for supplementation. When a person is sick, the bowel tolerance can increase by a factor of 100 times. So, a person with influenza, who in normal health would tolerate 2 grams a day, might consume 200 grams (200,000 mg) without any discomfort.

Strangely, the medical establishment classes the action of vitamin C on the bowel as an adverse side effect, but ignores the massive increase in bowel tolerance in the sick. Implausibly, a maximum recommended intake level has been set based on the smallest dose that might cause loose stools in some people. Given this, it is surprising that there are no government maximum recommended intakes for high-fiber foods such as beans. The U.S. Institute of Medicine had apparently decided that the intake of vitamin C must be limited, but could find no other side effects of large doses of vitamin C in healthy people. They set the maximum intake at 2 grams of vitamin C per day, as at this level almost no one in the population will suffer from diarrhea. Presumably, people have insufficient common sense to notice diarrhea and reduce their own intake. Despite several decades of attempts to find a reason why taking high doses of vitamin C could be harmful, detractors have not found toxicity simply because it does not exist.

CHAPTER 4

Conventional Medicine vs. Vitamin C

"A wealth of information creates a poverty of attention."
—HERBERT SIMON, *COMPUTERS, COMMUNICATIONS AND THE PUBLIC INTEREST*

Limitations of Social Medicine

The use of social medicine to investigate the actions and properties of vitamin C has inflamed and prolonged the controversy. To investigate heart disease, epidemiologists might look at how many people have heart attacks and determine the characteristics of people who are prone to the disease—for example, middle aged, overweight men, who smoke and eat junk food low in vitamin C. An epidemiologist can then determine the factors, such as environment, job hazards, family patterns, and personal habits that are more prevalent in people with coronary thrombosis. However, what epidemiology lacks is a high degree of explanatory power. To explain how a heart attack happens requires physics, biochemistry, and physiology. Without a grounding in these basics, epidemiology can degenerate into what some people have described as pseudoscience.[1]

An awareness of the limitations of epidemiology gives some perspective when considering the conflicting nutritional advice for good health, such as the requirements for vitamin C. According to popular myth, epidemiology "proved" that smoking causes lung cancer. Population studies certainly alerted scientists to the link between smoking and lung cancer, but this may have given an incorrect impression of the power of the statistical approach. A number of factors need to be in place before epidemiology can identify a potential causative agent.

We can be confident that cigarettes cause lung cancer, but epidemiology played only a small part in the justification. Most importantly, we have a detailed scientific explanation of how smoking causes lung cancer. Burning tobacco releases chemicals that cause genetic mutations, chromosome damage, irritation, and proliferation of cells, as well as oxidation of vitamin C.[2] The act of smoking delivers cancer-forming chemicals (carcinogens) to the delicate tissues of the lung and into the blood; they are found throughout the body tissues and are excreted in urine.[3] These chemicals have been observed to promote cancer in animal models,[4] although it can be difficult to reproduce the disease in healthy animals.[5] However, if animals with spontaneous tumors are forced to smoke, they develop increased numbers of lung tumors.[6] Thus, from our knowledge of basic pharmacology and biochemistry, the act of smoking can be predicted to increase the incidence of lung and other cancers.

Epidemiology points the way, giving an indication that a relationship between smoking and cancer exists, but by itself it does not provide a scientific explanation for that relationship. Given enough factors (or perhaps enough epidemiologists), spurious relationships can always be found. For example, since 1950, the number of televisions has increased in line with the level of carbon dioxide in the atmosphere. Can we conclude, therefore, that carbon dioxide causes televisions? The answer is clearly "no"—an example of the statistical rule that "correlation does not imply causation." In common language, just because two factors occur together does not necessarily mean that one causes the other.

Hill's Rules

Bradford Hill and Edward Kennaway, of St. Bartholomew's Hospital, London, investigated the epidemiology of smoking and lung cancer in 1947. Richard Doll joined the investigation slightly later. Doll later became a consultant to chemical and asbestos companies, who funded his research. His findings were highly criticized for underestimating the harm such products caused.[7] Ultimately, Doll's reputation suffered when this commercial involvement and potential bias was exposed, but Hill is regarded as having been "the world's leading medical statistician."[8]

It is perhaps sobering to remember that, at the time, smoking was common and few believed it could be associated with the disease. Reportedly, however, the Germans had already identified smoking as a cause of cancer.[9] Over the next forty years, it became apparent that smoking twenty-five or more cigarettes a day increased the risk of lung cancer by twenty-five times while lowering bodily reserves of vitamin C.[10] We can now state clearly that smoking tobacco promotes cancer, because, in addition to the epidemiology, we have an explanation of the processes involved from the basic physics, chemistry, and physiology.

Hill was aware of the limitations of epidemiology—unless the statistics are rigorously applied and the limitations of the data openly exposed, epidemiology can mislead more often than it informs. For this reason, Hill provided a set of criteria or rules that must be met before a causal link could be inferred.

- Plausibility: The measured correlation must be biologically plausible and there must be a rational, theoretical explanation for the phenomenon. This rule means that epidemiology (indeed, all clinical sciences) should conform to the underlying physiology and biochemistry.

- Strength of association: The observed relationship or correlation must be strong. Weak relationships constitute feeble evidence. Unfortunately, many medical claims on chronic illness and nutrition are based on weak relationships, such as the link between dietary cholesterol and heart disease. This rule might be taken as a caution against relationships that are commonly expressed as "percentage risk." It could also be another way of saying that if you need an enormous population to detect an effect, then that effect is probably too small to worry about.

- Timing: The proposed cause should precede the effect; also, the effect should be consistent with time. If the consumption of a substance varies over the years, then so should the associated disease. If the cause is removed and reintroduced, then the effect should vary.

- Dose-response relationship: The effect should increase with the intake or dose of the proposed causal factor (the more exposure to the substance, the greater should be the measured effect). We might add that the results should not be extrapolated outside the range of doses covered in the trial. This is a critical error in trials of vitamin C, where the dose employed is often less than 1 percent of the intake claimed to be effective. We will see how misrepresentation of dose levels has led to medicine's failure to investigate the claims for vitamin C and the common cold.

- Consistency: The relationship should be consistent when trials are repeated. The idea may be considered weak or even abandoned if subsequent results refute the suggestion. This rule suggests that the finding needs to be replicated, which is the basis of the scientific method.

- Coherence: The claimed effect must be consistent with scientific knowledge and should not conflict with other theories. If someone else has an alternative idea, it may provide a better explanation.

- Analogy: A commonly accepted phenomenon in one area can sometimes be used in another. The levels of ascorbic acid in animals that synthesize the vitamin are equivalent to an intake of several grams a day for a human. By analogy, the range of vitamin C intakes studied should encompass these doses but it seldom does.

- Experimental evidence: A proposed relationship should be shown independently, by experiment. Supporting experimental evidence from biochemistry, physics, or physiology greatly increases the plausibility of the proposed link.

- Singular cause: There should be only one cause rather than a list of risk factors. This final requirement is a blow to the proponents of multiple epidemiological risk factors for disease.

According to Hill, a pioneer of both the randomized clinical trial and epidemiology in medicine, all these criteria should be met before causation is assumed. Scientists in other disciplines might suggest that these conditions would be a minimal requirement for even a tentative indication of a causal relationship. These rules are basically common sense applied to data obtained from social and statistical studies of populations.

Epidemiology can be a powerful scientific tool, but it is often poorly applied. Hill's rules are rarely applied in modern epidemiology and the result is a continuous flood of apparently contradictory information. For example, in 1981, it was announced that coffee causes cancer of the pancreas and this might explain a large proportion of the cases in the United States.[11] Later, this well-publicized study was largely refuted.[12] Indeed, there are now indications that coffee might prevent other cancers.[13] True science tries to find underlying mechanisms and models explaining phenomena by cause and effect. Limitations of currently fashionable methods of medical investigation can severely hamper scientific progress.

Vitamin C and the Difficulties of Social Medicine

The increasing emphasis on risk factors and medicine as a social science can prevent proper investigation of the effects of vitamin C. Analysis of small, minimally effective doses has resulted in mixed findings and has spread confusion about ascorbate's true potential. The public release of such results leads to a gradual discrediting of the scientific method (misapplied epidemiology). Almost anything one does is supposedly implicated in one illness or another, causing anxiety and confusion in the minds of the public. Most people's vitamin C intake is low and population studies are based on these intakes. The high doses that might be effective in disease prevention are rarely investigated. Consequently, clinical trials and epidemiology are unlikely to show a clear link with vitamin C, even if shortage of it caused the disease.

Over the last half century, vitamin C studies have separated into those that investigate large doses and conventional research limited to micronutrient intakes. A factor central to the establishment's misrepresentation of the role of vitamin C has been the rise of social medicine, the idea that disease is a product of our social activities. An epidemiologist studies the population to investigate the habits of people and to contrast the diseased with the healthy. In one study, people with heart disease may have consumed more animal fat, a second study suggests lack of vitamins C or E, while another investigation implicates sugar. Subjects like environmental biology and ecology have the reputation for being soft sciences. However, the very nature of these subjects involves complexity and it can be hard to make simplifications and obtain general laws. When Charles Darwin claimed that "I am turned into a sort of machine for observing facts and grinding out conclusions," he was describing a particular form of genius that cannot be replaced by statistical analysis.

The design of accurate epidemiological studies presents great difficulty.[14] The first problem with epidemiology is choosing what factors are to be measured. This is a fundamental problem, not appreciated by many researchers. The problem of having a large group of potential factors is given a highly descriptive name in decision science—the curse of dimensionality. Paradoxically, beyond a certain point, using more factors decreases the predictive accuracy of the statistics: the more individual measures a study includes, the less accurate will be the result.

Suppose we wish to find dietary factors, such as vitamin C, that might relate to heart disease. There are thousands of potential candidates, from apples to zinc. Measuring each of these has an associated cost, as well as presenting practical difficulties. It is hard to determine accurately how much salt 10,000 people each consume over a period of a year, for example. It is clearly impractical to sample and measure every item in an individual's diet. Even if the population were highly constrained—for example, just soldiers consuming army food—the problems remain. Even soldiers have a choice of the food that they actually eat. Soldier A might hate broccoli, but could have a sweet tooth and love apple pie, whereas Soldier B never eats dessert but gets a food package every month from his family.

Often a researcher's solution is to simply ask the subjects what they eat by questionnaire and then to estimate the amounts of component nutrients from standard tables. For example, the investigator might assume an apple weighs 100 grams and contains 25 mg of vitamin C. However, even in this case that is apparently easy to estimate, values are subject to large errors. Apples come in different sizes and varieties, and they are stored for varying periods and subject to dissimilar treatments and methods of transport. Some are organic while others are mass-produced, and the amount of vitamin C in fruits and vegetables varies widely. Moreover, a subject reporting one apple a day may be confused, have a poor memory, or simply be lying.

The Framingham Study is one of the biggest medical investigations of the twentieth century and was highly influential on the growth of social medicine.[15] Before Framingham, clinical investigations of disease tended to be small or descriptive case reports.[16] Framingham began with support from the newly created U.S. National Heart Institute and the initial report of this long-term study, published in 1961, covered the first six years of following risk factors in the development of heart disease.[17] The results suggested that high blood pressure, smoking, and high cholesterol levels were in some way associated with heart disease. These risk factors emerged, but provided little insight into the disease. The follow-up has continued and over fifty years of data collected from Framingham residents has helped generate over 1,000 scientific papers.[18]

Framingham identified some risks associated with heart disease and stroke, but it also created a revolution in medicine by changing the way we view the origins of disease. It is claimed that the Framingham research dispelled the myth of a single cause of heart disease and started the now popular concept of risk factors. The results persuaded many researchers to concentrate on these risk factors instead of looking for a direct cause of the disease, such as chronic scurvy.[19] Unfortunately, Framingham data do not provide information that can help decide whether heart disease is a result of long-term vitamin C deficiency.

Back to Basic Science

History illustrates how medicine can go wrong by concentrating on epidemiology and clinical trials at the expense of primary scientific methods. In the nineteenth century, doctors attributed tuberculosis (TB), known as consumption or the white plague, to a combination of heredity or constitutional factors together with the miasma, or smells, in the environment. These risk factors, which seemed to explain how the disease was found to run in families, were thought to be the cause of TB.

It is easy to feel smug in the hindsight we have due to the benefit of accruing scientific knowledge. We now know that tuberculosis is a result of an infection that can lie dormant for years. There is a higher risk of contagion in confined spaces. Poorly nourished people with a low vitamin C intake, living in the same house as a TB sufferer, would have a greatly increased probability of catching the disease. With tuberculosis, the risk factors were a byproduct of the infectious process, but were mistaken as causes.

Bacteria cause tuberculosis, and it was Robert Koch who described the bacillus causing TB, *Mycobacterium tuberculosis,* in 1882. *Mycobacterium tuberculosis* is a slow-growing, aerobic bacterium that can divide every 16–20 hours. Koch discovered the cause of TB in the laboratory, after developing a new technique to stain the bacteria for microscopic identification. He won the Nobel Prize in Physiology or Medicine in 1905 for this discovery. Koch's success illustrates how disease mechanisms are discovered using basic biological science rather than social medicine. By concentrating on basic experimental science, Koch was able to demonstrate the single primary cause. Once the cause was understood, it explained the association with the risk factors.

John Snow, a London doctor, is sometimes described as the father of epidemiology. However, Snow's work on the London cholera epidemic in the 1850s was based on a new, theoretical understanding of the cause of disease. In the mid-nineteenth century, the primary risk factor for infection was thought to be bad smells. The name malaria, literally meaning "bad air," comes from this idea and remains as the modern name for the mosquito-borne disease. It is easy to see how infection was associated with bad smells—drinking contaminated malodorous water might cause disease and infected wounds would often release a putrid smell. While doctors assumed that bad smells caused infectious diseases like cholera, Snow's approach was an early form of germ theory.[20]

This led him to stop an outbreak of cholera in London.[21] By tracing the number of local cholera victims on a map, Snow noticed an association with a local well in Broad Street, Soho. Other people also produced maps of infection, using the data to support the miasma theory of disease.[22] Patients with the disease were marked with spots on the maps. More than fifty years before Snow, Valentine Seaman had used so-called spot maps to report deaths from yellow fever in New York.[23] Both the doctors who believed in contagion and their opponents used these maps to advance their respective causes.[24]

Snow's achievement arose because of his theoretical understanding of infection. His use of the map and "epidemiology" was to provide data to support his idea that special animal poisons spread infections. We now call these poisons "germs." The water in the Soho well was favored for its clarity and taste. For a doctor following the miasma theory of disease, it would be an unlikely place to look for the cause, because clear fresh water is odorless and thus inconsistent with the miasma theory of disease. Snow's adoption of the germ theory led him to make his discovery. He removed the pump from the well and the epidemic subsided.

Close to John Snow lived another pioneer in health, the engineer Joseph Bazalgette (1819–1891). Like Snow, Bazalgette was to lead the way in disease prevention and, arguably, he made the larger practical contribution. He designed and built the London sewers to rid the city of the intolerable smell and miasma of the river Thames, and thus prevent disease.[25] Sewers brought sanitation to London and, eventually, to the world. Serendipitously, Bazalgette's response to the miasma theory prevented the deaths of millions. Working from the unsound association of disease with bad smells, engineering may have saved more lives than any physician. Bazalgette's ultimate achievement came about through serendipity, a correct result based on faulty reasoning.

Today, we expect a response to illness based on solid scientific evidence and, particularly, the biological mechanisms underlying the disease. It is clearly insufficient to have a limited practical understanding based on risk factors and hope we end up, like Bazalgette, preventing disease by chance. Snow showed the way, not by mapping the disease, which was an established approach to following epidemics, but by utilizing his knowledge of disease mechanisms.

The mechanisms for the antiviral and anticancer actions of massive doses of vitamin C are already established.[26] When combined with clinical observations from physicians reporting remarkable effects, there is sufficient data to demand clinical trials. Snow's work was based on a new understanding of disease. But even now, people promoting the risk factor approach appropriate his success, describing him as the founding father of modern epidemiology. In Snow's day, his germ-based ideas had few supporters compared with the miasma theory. Similarly, clinical trials of vitamin C in large doses do not fall within the mindset of current medical opinion, which is dominated by ideas of science as sociology.

Whenever medical problems and disease are described in terms of risk factors, the biological understanding is deficient. Finding new scientific explanations is difficult. It often relies on the ability of an individual scientist to see through the mess of risk factors in order to provide a simple model or theory. Most medical problems have a simple explanation. Shortage of vitamin C may be the underlying cause of heart disease, arthritis, and many other chronic conditions facing modern humans, but medicine's risk factor approach to studying disease today is unlikely to be able to confirm or refute this idea in the foreseeable future.

Limiting True Progress

Social science and genetics now have increasing preeminence in medicine to the detriment of true progress. This emphasis on social medicine is a relatively new phenomenon, popularized since the 1950s. Unfortunately, the further medicine gets from a physiological or biochemical understanding of disease, the less scientific progress is made. Since this new approach was adopted, medical progress on the leading causes of disease has slowed.

The idea that disease is a product of our social activities dominates current medicine. Social medicine is a pragmatic form of clinical science that downgrades the importance of theory, biochemistry, and physiology.

Large-scale studies have become a preferred form of research—identifying the relative importance of minor risk factors. While such detailed scientific information gathering from populations is useful, it can also constrain the progress of medical science. Scientific advancement typically depends on developing new theories based on interpretation of the physical evidence. A major advance in molecular biology in the latter half of the twentieth century was the double helix model for the structure of DNA, which resulted from the work of Rosalind Franklin, Frances Crick, and James D. Watson in the early 1950s. This simple theory enabled rapid advances to be made in genetics and cell biology. Currently, however, medicine seems to abhor biological theory and understanding, preferring to study statistical relationships between social influences, risk factors, and disease. Such science fails to describe the mechanisms involved. Consequently, the understanding needed to solve medical problems becomes increasingly difficult to achieve.

Practical medicine is a craft rather than science, and in the hands of the more accomplished doctors, it might even be called an art. However, it is art constrained by scientific principles and facts. Social science can be practical and helpful, but it is not normally considered a hard science. A clinical trial, for example, is a direct measure of the performance of a treatment and can suggest whether the treatment will be useful in practice, but a clinical trial is unlikely to help scientists understand the underlying pharmacology or pathology associated with the disease. When practical ideas, culture, and current practice are allowed to dominate the field of medicine, innovation and advancement are slowed. Big advances, such as Alexander Fleming's discovery of penicillin in 1928, typically arise from observation and experiment.

The Search for "Proof"

The conventional model for good health is one in which people take regular exercise, have a diet low in fat and salt, and get their vitamin C from five daily helpings of fruit and vegetables. According to the authorities, vitamin C supplementation is unnecessary if a person eats a normal, healthy diet. Governments parade these recommendations as scientific facts. However, people who conform to these standard "healthy" recommendations can still have low vitamin C levels, get cancer, or die prematurely of heart disease. It may be that non-smoking vegetarians who exercise will die a little less prematurely, but that is hardly comforting to the majority.

People are getting fatter, eating more junk food, and taking less exercise, but, paradoxically, since the 1950s, deaths from cardiovascular disease have been falling. This recent lowering of mortality often comes as a surprise to those who rely on the popular media for information. The well-publicized risk factors, such as cholesterol, do not explain the rise and fall of heart disease in the twentieth century.[27] People are bombarded with helpful information, though often it is conflicting. Mostly, it is well-meaning but based on weak evidence. The experts providing the advice often ensure that it meets currently accepted practice or, at least, is consistent with the prevailing ideas. Frequently, such advice is described as scientifically proven. By contrast, alternative medicine is portrayed as unproven. Epidemiology, supported by clinical trials, underlies these claims of scientific proof.

The finding that people with lung cancer often smoke cigarettes typifies the popular description of medical "proof." This form of association may occasionally be useful in generating a new scientific hypothesis or be helpful in confirming a scientific finding, but it does not constitute proof.

In the first half of the last century, medical science made great strides, with the discovery of insulin for diabetes and antibiotics for infections, the beginnings of molecular biology, and advances in surgery. Since then, progress has slowed dramatically, with fewer groundbreaking therapies. Many recent advances are imports from other disciplines. X-ray computed tomography and magnetic resonance imaging have come from physics, for example. Sciences related to medicine, including biochemistry and genetics, have made steady progress, but this has not yet translated into revolutionary new medical treatments with high impacts on the major diseases.

James Le Fanu, M.D., author of *The Rise and Fall of Modern Medicine,* suggests that the introduction of social medicine, together with a gene-centric approach to disease, has caused this lack of progress. Medicine has stopped looking at the important data, such as the observations of Frederick R. Klenner, M.D., on the effect of massive doses of vitamin C, relying instead on indirect measures and statistics. It is as if medical science has lost the knack of finding cures for disease. By becoming dominated by the search for "proof," medicine is giving up the scientific method. Science is a search for the explanation of how things work, not a search for something called "proof" that, by direct implication, prevents questioning. The repeated use of the term *proof* in medicine carries within it the suggestion of "cargo cult" science, a form of pseudo-science that has all the trappings of real science and appears to follow its rules, but is ineffective (or at least very inefficient) at expanding the knowledge base.

"Cargo Cult" Science

In 1974, the physicist Richard Feynman, Ph.D., described a phenomenon that he called "cargo cult" science.[28] At that time, the magician Uri Geller had gained prominence for his claims of bending spoons, keys, and other inanimate objects with the power of his mind alone. The idea came to Dr. Feynman when Geller had been unable to demonstrate his key bending skills for Dr. Feynman to investigate. Powerless to evaluate Geller's claim directly, he wondered why witch doctors had managed to practice for so long when a simple check on their performance would have exposed them.

Dr. Feynman remembered the South Seas people who developed what became known as a "cargo cult." In the Second World War, airplanes brought goods and materials to the islands, landing on temporary airfields. After the war, when the planes no longer arrived, the islanders tried to reproduce the phenomenon by making new runways with small fires alongside. This provided a close approximation to what had been there before. A wooden hut for a man to sit in, wearing headphones with bamboo antennas, improved the illusion. The representation was excellent, but airplanes still did not land. However, even though scheduled flights would never land, a pilot in trouble from mechanical failure or fuel shortage might take advantage of the pseudo-airfield. Thus, the runway had reduced the risk that no future landings would occur.

The missing item in cargo cult science, according to Dr. Feynman, is scientific integrity. Scientists should always be looking out for data that does not fit. Such data explain how limited and tenuous ideas are. When alternative explanations are compatible with the data, scientists acknowledge the correspondence. The last thing a good scientist does is describe their work as scientific "proof." By analogy, cargo cult science, based on a multitude of risk factors and asserting "proof," looks like science, but it is not real understanding.

Scientifically, it is not possible to prove anything—science does not work like that. A scientist has an idea, called a hypothesis, such as the idea that massive doses of vitamin C can destroy cancer. The scientist then attempts to disprove or refute this idea by experimenting or by finding counter examples, and the idea may be modified in the light of new data. This process continues until the idea is shown to be wrong and can be replaced by an alternative. This approach, in its modern form, is derived from the philosopher Karl Popper. However, the method is somewhat similar in form to the Socratic method in philosophy, which involves *elenchus*, a cross-examination for the purpose of refutation. In practice, scientists use loose reasoning and inference to generate new ideas. If an experimental result does not come out quite as expected, there might be an alternative explanation. Experiments test these ideas, which may prove correct or may be rejected. This process of getting ideas, testing them, and throwing them away when they do not work is very powerful and has provided humanity with its expanding scientific knowledge.

A vital feature of cargo cult science is the lack of explanation. In a real airport, the controller's headphones receive radio signals from the aircraft. This is described by basic physics, providing a rationalization for the artifact on the controller's head. No such justification comes with the use of bamboo headphones, no matter how well-made or how closely they resemble the originals. When doctors started searching for patterns of risk and downgrading the underlying scientific mechanisms, medicine adopted the practice of cargo cult science.

The Misrepresentation of Vitamin C

There is much excitement about "evidence-based medicine" as a relatively new initiative, but this is not an indication of a scientific discipline. A corresponding phrase such as "evidence-based physics" sounds oddly ridiculous.[35] Physics is a rigorous science and the idea that part of physics is based on evidence implies that some physics is not based on evidence, which seems absurd. The term *evidence-based medicine* is an indication that medical science is in a bad way.

As we were writing this book, the media was filled with stories about vitamin C being ineffective against the common cold. Headlines included "Vitamin C Useless for Preventing or Treating Colds," "C Branded the World's Most Pathetic Vitamin," and "Vitamin C Nearly Useless vs. Colds." The tumult followed a minor update to an earlier Cochrane review, which

Peptic Ulcers and the Concept of "Proof"

The example of peptic ulcers illustrates the pernicious effects of "proof" in medicine. The concept that something can be proven in science is not only wrong, but stifles progress. For example, if doctors believe it has been proven that stress causes stomach ulcers, there is no point in looking elsewhere for a better explanation. For years, it was understood that stress caused acid in the stomach, which led to peptic ulcers. People with ulcers were asked to modify their diet to include foods that made the stomach more alkaline. A basic medication was calcium carbonate, otherwise known as chalk, which would buffer stomach acid.

There was a substantial amount of data relating increased acidity in the stomach to gastritis (inflammation) and the eventual formation of ulcers. For this reason, the proposal that increased acid in the stomach could be an irritant, leading to damage, appeared obvious. The idea that excess acid in the stomach was the cause of ulcers reached a peak when the drug Cimetidine was introduced in 1976. Receptors for histamine, a local hormone associated with inflammation, were discovered in the stomach and were associated with acidity and increased risk of ulceration. Cimitedine and related drugs block these receptors, lowering stomach acid.

When medicine does not fully understand the physiology and pathology of an illness, it often relegates it to a psychological effect.[29] People under stress were thought more likely to suffer from peptic ulcers, and animal studies provided additional support for the link.[30] In humans, white collar workers (who were strangely assumed to be highly stressed) had the disease more frequently than manual workers did. The explanation appeared clear-cut with little reason for a scientific challenge. In recent times, a researcher might have assumed that the decades of study into this common disease had provided "proof" that stress and increased acid causes peptic ulcers. Standard physiology textbooks stated as a fact that the cause of peptic ulcer in humans was stress.[31]

In the early 1980s, Dr. Robin Warren of the Royal Perth Hospital, in Western Australia, found bacteria in specimens from people with chronic gastritis. Gastritis or inflammation of the stomach often happens when stomach ulcers are developing. The bacteria occurred in about half the specimens and in numbers that should have been evident on routine examination. However, these small bacteria appeared to be new to pathologists and were later given the name *Helicobacter pylori*. These previously unknown bacteria were in the stomachs of the majority of people suffering gastritis and ulcers. A course of antibiotics removed the bacteria, along with the ulceration and gastritis.

Helicobacter is now an accepted cause of peptic ulcer and antibiotics are a standard treatment.[32] Even a low-carbohydrate diet can prevent and reverse heartburn and gastritis in many people.[33] Notably, the medical establishment did not accept these findings for a number of years. The conventional explanation is that medicine is conservative and requires substantial verification before findings can become recommended therapy. More cynically, the histamine drugs like Cimetidine were still profitably under patent—they came off prescription and were available over the counter during the period in which *H. pylori* gained slow acceptance.

The discovery that peptic ulcer was an infectious disease has eventually been turned into a success story for modern medicine. Scientific disasters may be transformed into triumphs given sufficient time and hype. In this case, the level of incompetence was astounding. A major disease, which was relatively easy to study, was misunderstood for decades. Any doctor or pathologist examining stomach tissue could have sampled and identified the offending bacteria. This failure of medical science is clearly a result of relying on indirect evidence and not examining the disease mechanism. The concept of "proof" has no place in science, stifles innovation, and protects vested interests.[34]

contained little extra information and no new conclusions, but the insignificant update generated negative publicity throughout the world.[36] The Cochrane Collaboration is an international not-for-profit organization dedicated to making up-to-date health-care information readily available. It claims to provide a gold standard in evidence-based medical studies, but prejudice and bias against vitamin C has invaded even that organization. We will look at the Cochrane study on vitamin C and the common cold as an example of medical pseudo-science.

It's All About the Dose

The intakes of vitamin C required to prevent colds are often misunderstood. The dose-response relationship is fundamental to pharmacology: most biological responses vary with dose size. This finding is so firmly established that it barely requires repeating. However, Harri Hemilä and colleagues, who compiled the Cochrane review, apparently believe they can break the basic laws of pharmacology by using statistics.

The original findings by Frederick R. Klenner, M.D., and others were

for doses of vitamin C in the region of 10 grams or more, which prevented colds in most people. Hemilä's study considered doses above 200 mg,
which is only 2 percent of Dr. Klenner's minimum dose. The Cochrane
review included three dose intervals: between 200 mg and 1 gram per day,
between 1 and 2 grams per day, and above 2 grams per day. However,
there were only three prevention studies with more than 2 grams a day,
and each used a dose of only 3 grams.[37]

Some proponents of evidence-based medicine appear to think a good
trial is one that obeys a specific recipe in the way it is conducted. The
recipe specifies the study must be randomized with placebo controls. In
the Cochrane review of vitamin C, the studies did not reach the minimum
intake claimed to be effective at preventing the common cold.[38] The
Cochrane review, however, bizarrely considered that Linus Pauling's vig-
orous advocacy for vitamin C was the stimulus for a wave of "good trials," meaning randomized, placebo-controlled clinical trials as opposed to
well-designed experiments that actually addressed the doses of vitamin C
claimed to be effective. Cochrane claims these trials enabled a better
understanding of the role that vitamin C plays in defense against the common cold. However, we would be extremely surprised if Dr. Pauling would
have considered these so-called good trials relevant to the use of high-dose
vitamin C against the common cold.

The review included doses that were both inappropriate and inadequate,
with no account for the rules of pharmacology. No data were provided to
indicate whether doses above 3 grams per day could be effective for preventing the common cold. Despite this, in the Cochrane report's conclusions, data for 3 grams or less were applied to vitamin C in general,
regardless of the dose. Consider, as an analogy, a study of the effects of
Scotch whisky. As is well known, a glass of whisky will warm, two glass-
es may make a person tipsy, but a bottle or two can kill. If the Cochrane
study had investigated the use of whisky, the author might have reviewed
studies in which people consumed up to a fifth of a glass. Since no subjects became tipsy, the review would conclude that reports of people
becoming drunk on alcohol were clearly a myth. Headlines around the
world might have declared "Whisky Useless as an Intoxicant!"

If the doses claimed to prevent the common cold are large, those used
to treat it are massive. A gram or two of vitamin C will have almost no
effect on an existing cold or similar infection. This is not in dispute. The

people reinforcing this suggestion are trying to discredit the use of high doses and, as we have explained, 1 gram of vitamin C is not a large dose. Robert F. Cathcart III, M.D., has observed that people can take much more vitamin C when they have a cold.[39] Typical healthy people can take between 4 and 15 grams of vitamin C a day before reaching bowel tolerance. For a person with a mild cold, the tolerance goes up to between 30 and 60 grams. A severe cold produces an even greater increase, in the region of 60 to 100 grams, or more.[40] Dr. Cathcart suggests up to fifteen divided doses per day to produce a sustained intake.[41]

The Cochrane study does not address these dosages, but uses small intakes for treatment as well as prevention. The largest dose of vitamin C in the Cochrane study was about ten times smaller than those claimed to provide an effective treatment. Hemilä and colleagues make much of the inclusion of a study that used a single 8-gram dose at the beginning of a cold, which they claim provided "equivocal benefit." However, another study included a comparison of doses of 4 grams and 8 grams given on the first day of illness.[42] The average duration of illness in the 4-gram group was 3.17 days, while in those receiving 8 grams this was reduced to 2.86 days, a significant result. These results suggest that the effect of a single dose of 8 grams is larger than the response for 4 grams. Despite the fact that a single 8-gram dose would not normally be considered sufficient for treatment, these results are consistent with repeated clinical observations of benefit for massive doses of vitamin C.

Most people understand that a low dose of a drug may be used to prevent a disease. When the disease becomes established, the dose of the drug needs to be increased with the severity of the illness. Antibiotics provide an example: a low oral dose of antibiotic could be used to prevent infection, but if the person becomes ill, it is necessary to increase the dose. In the Cochrane study, the dose-response relationship of vitamin C is apparently considered irrelevant.

Pharmacokinetics

The study of how a drug is absorbed, distributed in the body, and excreted is known as pharmacokinetics. Some substances are poorly absorbed and this may have advantages; for example, magnesium oxide is occasionally used to prevent constipation. Other substances, such as high doses of vitamin C, are rapidly excreted. In understanding the action of a drug or nutrient, it is essential to appreciate the way it is absorbed and excreted.

Drugs and nutrients often interact and bind to protein molecules called receptors, which fit their shape as a key matches a lock. The biological effect depends on the proportion of receptors occupied. If the concentration is low, few receptors are occupied and the response is correspondingly small. As the local drug concentration increases, more is bound to the receptors and the biological effect is greater. At high doses, practically all the receptors are occupied, producing a maximum response. Most drug reactions and many nutrient effects are explained in this way.

Vitamin C interacts with receptors on enzymes and other proteins. However, ascorbate also acts as an antioxidant. When acting as an antioxidant, it donates electrons and the number of electrons available depends on the amount of vitamin C present. The actions of vitamin C are highly dose-dependent and somewhat unusual. For example, low doses of vitamin C are retained in the body and have an effective half-life of somewhere between eight and forty days. By contrast, high doses are excreted many hundreds of times more rapidly. Thus, it is not possible to predict the effects of a large dose using data from a low dose.

We previously mentioned the contraceptive pill as an example of the importance of dose frequency. Contraception usually involves taking a single dose, once a day, through the monthly cycle. The entire month's supply cannot be given as a single large dose at the start of the month, because such a large dose may have toxic effects and may be ineffective. Moreover, the hormones are expected to be removed from the blood rapidly. In order to be effective as contraceptives, the pill needs to be taken on a daily basis. Women complaining that they became pregnant after missing just one or two pills are describing a process that can be predicted from pharmacokinetics. Missing doses means the blood levels return to baseline in a short interval and the molecular receptors inhibiting pregnancy are no longer occupied. Few doctors would be surprised if women not taking the pill regularly became pregnant.

The excretion half-life of vitamin C is short, so a single tablet will not raise blood levels for more than a few hours. For the rest of the day, blood levels will fall back to the baseline. However, the Cochrane review on vitamin C and the common cold takes no account of the dose interval. Expecting a single, daily gram-level dose of vitamin C to prevent a cold is equivalent to a woman expecting to prevent pregnancy with just one pill a month. The Cochrane review expects vitamin C to work when it is not present in the body. For example, a person taking a gram of vitamin C in the morning may have baseline levels by the afternoon, when she travels home from work and takes her bus ticket from the hand of a cold-infected driver. The virus will enter her body and multiply during the evening and throughout the night. Her plasma vitamin C levels will drop. By the following morning, when she takes another gram of vitamin C, the virus will be well established and growing. The dose may not even raise her blood levels back to baseline and will have little or no effect on the progress of the cold.

The Cochrane Review—"Cargo Cult" Science?

The Cochrane review suggests that massive doses used to treat the common cold can be discounted. Of the reports from Dr. Cathcart and other independent physicians, they say that "their uncontrolled observations do not provide valid evidence of benefit." Here, we enter a topsy-turvy world, where logic is inadmissible. To the physicians who compiled the Cochrane study, repeated, direct observation and measurement by multiple independent researchers is not only less important than a single clinical trial, it provides no valid evidence at all.

The Cochrane approach indicates that there is apparently no valid evidence that there was a volcanic eruption at Mount St. Helens on May 18, 1980. You may have seen the television record, read it in the newspaper, or perhaps you witnessed it yourself. You may know of scientists who measured the earth tremors, or sampled, measured, and chemically analyzed the rock ejected from the mountain. You may have copies of satellite images that independently recorded and measured the event. However, to the Cochrane Collaboration, these data are irrelevant and provide no valid evidence as they constitute uncontrolled observations.

While Cochrane's comments suggest that geologists have no valid evidence for the existence of volcanoes or earthquakes, other scientists are in even more trouble. Physics, with its basis of direct, repeatable observation and measurement, should have a new sub-discipline. We suggest the name evidence-based physics, where the only evidence considered valid comes from repeated statistical trials using the methods prescribed by the Cochrane Collaboration. Mathematics and logic may be ignored entirely.

In a summary clearly aimed at the public and press, the Cochrane study states, "Thirty trials involving 11,350 participants suggest that regular ingestion of vitamin C has no effect on common cold incidence in the ordinary population." This is a general statement implying that vitamin C supplementation, irrespective of dose or frequency, does not prevent the common cold. However, to support such a statement, the authors would need to demonstrate that they had tested the appropriate doses. They have not—the doses tested were far too small. The Vitamin C Foundation's advice is: "At first sign of cold or flu, begin taking at least 8 grams (8,000 mg) of vitamin C as ascorbic acid every twenty minutes for three to four hours until bowel tolerance. Continue with smaller dosages of 2–4 grams every 4–6 hours for ten days to prevent recurrence."[43]

Readers are asked to decide for themselves how much confidence they place in the Cochrane review of vitamin C and the common cold. We agree with Linus Pauling: people should "always be skeptical—always think for yourself." Efforts to produce evidence-based medicine can be counterproductive if they exclude valuable sources of information. Repeated, easily replicable observation provides, if anything, more direct and reliable evidence than clinical trials.

Tarnished Gold

Conventionally, the core requirement for medical "proof" consists of randomized, placebo-controlled clinical trials, a basic form of experiment for testing therapies on people. Any assertion of the effectiveness of vitamin C tends to be rebutted by a request to see the clinical trial data. As we have seen, all other evidence is effectively discounted. One leading physician even argued that the reports of the remarkable effectiveness of massive doses of vitamin C, by physicians such as Drs. Klenner and Cathcart, could simply be wishful thinking and the placebo effect. The only way to be sure would be to have clinical trials, but such clinical trials, which are fifty years overdue, are not in the works from any conventional scientists in the foreseeable future. Ironically, the medical establishment demands such evidence but withholds the funds that would make it possible—a perfect catch-22.

Clinical trials face public distrust, while the establishment continues to see this form of experiment as the "gold standard" for clinical medicine. Pharmaceutical companies see them as a form of advertising and increasingly dominate trials.[44] But the general public are skeptical of such clinical research and the majority of Americans do not trust research information from pharmaceutical companies.[45] As time passes, fewer people are willing to accept reported clinical trial results, falling from an estimated 72 percent in 1996 to 30 percent in 2002. Harris Interactive, a market research and polling firm, estimates that only 14 percent of Americans consider drug companies to be honest, a figure comparable to their opinion of the tobacco, oil, and used car industries.[46] Today, 70 percent of people believe that drug companies put profits ahead of patients' interests.[47] This should be expected of commercial companies, as profit is their reason for existence.

Knowledge should always be considered tentative. Even in the face of remarkable observations, such as dying children recovering within minutes of an ascorbate injection,[48] we need to be suitably skeptical. In reviewing the available evidence, it is essential to be aware of basic problems with scientific data. For example, some patients simply get better by themselves. Spontaneous remission is more common than people realize and can confound experimental results.[49] Demand characteristics are another problem: some patients report what they believe their doctors want to hear. A related effect, effort justification, is when patients feel the need to rationalize the effort and cost of treatment (for example, "This chemotherapy is so tough and expensive, it must be effective!"). However, the factor given most prominence in clinical trials is the placebo. But despite claims by conventional physicians, the placebo effect cannot be used to explain the clinical observations with massive doses of vitamin C.

The Powerful Placebo?

The classic and well-known placebo (Latin for "I shall please") effect occurs when patients expect to get better and their condition improves, irrespective of the treatment. Doctors assume this effect is so powerful that new drug treatments need to be tested against a dummy pill, in a so-called placebo-controlled trial. These trials are designed to make sure that at least some of the observed improvement is actually caused by the drug rather than the act of treating the patient.

Despite a widespread assumption that the placebo effect is valid, some scientists dispute its existence.[50] Numerous factors can cause an apparent placebo effect to arise in experimental data and several other mechanisms might explain placebo effects. Factors such as spontaneous improvement, fluctuation of symptoms, additional treatment, conditional switching of placebo treatment, irrelevant response variables, conditioned answers, neurotic or psychotic misjudgment, and psychosomatic phenomena could contribute to the bias described as the placebo effect. In a well-designed trial, use of a control group is a method to reduce sources of bias.

The placebo effect may be a result of psychological conditioning, a sort of trained response no matter what the treatment. Under this view, the reported effects of vitamin C might be explained as a placebo effect arising from a conditioned response to treatment. An alternative psychological description of the placebo response is the subject-expectancy effect, a bias that occurs when a subject expects a result and unconsciously manipulates an experiment or reports the expectation. This is similar to the observer-expectancy effect, which is when a researcher is expecting a result and unconsciously modifies an experiment, or misinterprets data, in order to find it. Experimenter bias leads to the use of double-blind clinical trials, when neither the experimenter nor the patient knows who is getting the treatment or the placebo until the experiment is concluded and the results are analyzed.

A placebo is an inert pill or substance with no pharmacological effect but which may have psychological therapeutic value. Others extend its meaning to cover any therapy or procedure that has no direct biochemical effect but that may induce a psychological response. The opposite effect, nocebo (Latin for "I shall harm"), is when a patient believes that a treatment will cause harm and experiences adverse side effects when given an inert substance.[51] The view of conventional medicine on vitamin C is that any benefit is attributed to the placebo effect, while minor (possibly nocebo) side effects are given great prominence.

The placebo effect is taken for granted in the design of most clinical trials, but the facts are somewhat different. Scientists have used controlled clinical trials to investigate the effectiveness of placebo against no treatment. Numerous trials to investigate the placebo effect have been performed, and an analysis of 130 such experiments was recently reported.[52] Strikingly, of the many studies investigated, none was able to distinguish between a placebo effect and the natural course of a disease. It seems that people recovering naturally from a disease can have their improvement attributed to the placebo effect. These experimental results suggest that the placebo effect is severely limited in terms of the physiological responses it can elicit.[53] Perhaps unexpectedly, the experimental data indicate that placebo controls are not important in trials of vitamin C with definitive outcomes. A definitive outcome would be the death of the patient, abrupt termination of symptoms, cure of the disease, or some other direct physical response. Sixteen of the 130 investigated trials of the placebo were excluded because they did not have sufficient data on outcomes. Definitive outcomes were present in 32 trials involving a total of 3,795 patients. These trials showed no placebo effect, irrespective of whether the outcome was subjective or objective.

The implications of these findings are clear. While the description of the placebo as a myth or a scam might be going too far, its effects have been grossly overestimated.[54] For example, attribution to the placebo effect would be a weak criticism for a study of treatment with vitamin C which produces a five-fold longer survival time in terminal cancer patients.[55] Stated simply, if a placebo were such an effective treatment for cancer, it would put current medical practice to shame.

In retrospect, these limitations of the placebo effect should be expected. Basic science and repeatable observation should take precedence over statistical evidence. Nonetheless, to evidence-based medicine, suggesting that a physical event, such as shooting a person through the heart, causes the death of the subject would be speculation. Apparently, it would be necessary to perform a randomized, placebo-controlled clinical trial to show the effectiveness of a physical barrier, such as a Kevlar bulletproof vest. We would need to show statistically that a greater number of people who were shot through the heart died compared with matched controls who wore the vest. Rationally, a bulletproof vest does not need to be compared with a sugar pill in preventing damage from a bullet—we understand the mechanisms involved and the results are definitive.

In the case of vitamin C and viral infections, the claimed effects of complete cessation of symptoms and "cure" are not achievable by any other substance or medication. With the common cold, the disease is generally mild and the discussion somewhat academic. However, modern medicine refuses the patient suffering from severe viral infection, or terminal cancer, the choice of a treatment with vitamin C. Given a disease with no effective alternative therapy and a safe treatment claimed to be highly effective with little risk, the rational decision is clear.

With subjective outcomes, a placebo can have a beneficial effect. Pain is highly subjective and continuous in character and, like psychiatric problems such as depression, might be expected to show a placebo response.[56] A continuous outcome is when the effect is scaled from minor to major responses: for example, a patient is asked to estimate the pain they are suffering on a scale of 1 to 10. The placebo effect may be biased toward smaller trials, as it appears to decrease with increasing numbers of patients. A larger number of smaller trials (82), with 4,730 patients in total, had continuous outcomes. The placebo was effective in subjective trials, as might be expected.[57] Notably, twenty-seven trials showing benefit from placebo involved the treatment of pain.

The placebo effect has little role in explaining the clinical observations of physicians administering massive doses of vitamin C. If the placebo could be an effective therapy against viral disease, as described for vitamin C by Drs. Klenner and Cathcart, we would not have to worry about such infections. Unfortunately, even the most powerful conventional antiviral medications are largely futile against severe viral diseases.

However, the markedly limited placebo effect is not a reason for minimizing the effect of brain states and psychology in medicine. While the placebo effect is overestimated, the potential of psychological medicine is often underestimated. There is more to psychological medicine than the humble placebo. Nevertheless, it is compelling to compare conventional medicine's over-ready acceptance of claims for the not-so-powerful placebo with its response to the clinical observations on vitamin C of Drs. Klenner, Cathcart, and Stone.

Random Trials

The randomized, placebo-controlled trial is considered the gold standard of clinical evidence, leading to its cult status in medicine.[58] However, without the support of basic science from physiology, pharmacology, and biochemistry, the utility of the clinical trial is severely limited. With little modification, Bradford Hill's requirements for epidemiology are applicable when considering clinical trials. Clinical trials are merely a technique for measuring the practical value of a therapy, but over-emphasis on the importance of clinical trials devalues information from other sources, such as natural history studies, clinical experience, and case reports. Over the years, evidence for the benefits of vitamin C from these sources has accumulated. While the randomized, controlled trial is important as a practical measure, it is not the only source of scientific information.

Choosing patients for a clinical trial is always a problem. Each person is biologically unique and has an individual response to diseases and treatment.[59] Even unconscious bias in choosing patients for an experiment can give invalid results. To reduce the potential for bias, patients in clinical trials are often randomly assigned to the treatment group or the control group. However, effective randomization is difficult to achieve in practice. For example, a suitable criterion is needed for the random selection, such as the order of presentation at the clinic. Even when the groups are fully random, people leaving the study can reintroduce bias. In selective attrition, patients who do not benefit from a treatment or who suffer side effects may drop out, leaving a more positive group of subjects.

Many trials match people in the two randomly selected groups—both groups may be additionally chosen to have a narrow age range or, alternatively, an equal number of males and females in each group. Random selection might otherwise lead, for example, to two sex-biased groups of twelve patients, with four females in one group and ten in the other. Alternatively, a randomly selected treatment group with an average age of seventy-five could have a randomly selected control group of teenagers. These are extreme examples with obvious differences easily noted by the researchers, but since the number of characteristics to match is very large, randomization could easily leave two groups which differ in many unmatched features (blood type, for example). Background knowledge of the underlying disease processes can suggest important characteristics to match in a particular study. Despite this matching, the groups in randomized, controlled clinical trials are substantially different biologically.

A Mean Regression

One strange and not fully explained phenomenon of clinical trials is that the first time an experiment is done, the results can be excellent, but subsequent experiments produce less dramatic improvements with the treatment. This trend is a form of regression to the mean, in which extreme results tend to become more average over time. Regression to the mean can result in wrongly concluding that an effect is due to treatment when it is due to chance. It is also an explanation of how the data from clinical trials can apparently support the existence of the placebo effect.[60] A group of people selected for a clinical trial is not representative of the population but biased, by definition, as they are sick. Often patients will get better with time, or regress to the mean, over the period of the trial. In most trials, regression will be indistinguishable from a placebo effect.

In 1886, British statistician Francis Galton (1822–1911), a half cousin of Charles Darwin, first described "regression towards mediocrity," which now has the more politically correct name of regression to the mean.[61] Galton measured the height of adults and their parents. When the parents' height was greater than average, the children were shorter than the parents. However, when the parents were shorter than average, the children tended to be taller than their parents. Flight instructors provide a more recent example: when instructors praised a trainee pilot for an excellent landing, typically their next landing attempt was poor.[62] It is easy to see how the instructors thought that praising the trainees was counterproductive, but the real explanation was regression toward the mean.[63]

In some studies, patients diagnosed with a particular disease may have another malady or could even be healthy.[64] Clinical diagnosis can be subjective. In these cases, the experiment can give completely misleading results, as the subjects do not even have the disease being considered. Another source of error arises when patients receive more than one treatment at a time and the therapies interact.[65] The results obtained could result from any one of the therapies or from some interaction between them. This multiple treatment interference is not easy to disentangle from the raw data obtained in an experiment and is a more particular problem when a large number of variables are considered.

Unreliable Results

The justification of both clinical trials and epidemiology is based largely on statistics, but many clinical studies provide unbelievable statistical results. Peter Gøtzsche, of the Nordic Cochrane Centre and Network, recently investigated statistics in clinical trials published in 2003.[66] He found that many of the reported data were potentially biased. The results were calculated from small selections of the subjects studied or were derived from a biased collection of results. These potentially prejudiced results were reported without explanation in 98 percent of 260 trials. Gøtzsche was able to check the calculations for twenty-seven of the trials and found that a quarter of all results deemed "non-significant" were actually significant. Furthermore, four of the twenty-three reportedly significant results were wrong, five were doubtful, and another four were open to interpretation.

Significant results in abstracts should generally be disbelieved. Abstracts of papers are often the only section read in detail and frequently contain unsupported data.[67] When a new drug is studied, the bias typically presents the drug in a more positive light. For example, in all but one of eighty-two studies, bias in the conclusion or abstract of comparative trials of two anti-inflammatory drugs consistently favored the new drug over the control drug.[68] Based on this information, doctors might prefer to prescribe a profitable new drug when it actually has no benefit over existing medicine.

Many clinical trials are designed to produce significant results. A large number of statistical tests are often built into the trials. Indeed, trials which include more than 200 statistical tests are sometimes specified in protocols.[69] A trial with 200 tests of identical drugs is almost certain to produce one or more significant results by chance alone. Thus, statistically significant improvements will be reported for a new drug even if it was identical to the one with which it was compared. By boosting the number of tests, a drug company can be fairly certain that it will get a result that will be useful for marketing the drug.

Additional measures are sometimes used to massage clinical results. Studies comparing study designs with the actual published reports of clinical trials have revealed selective use of data to overestimate the effectiveness of the treatment.[70] This selective reporting bias occurs even in "high quality" government-funded studies.[71] As a result, the medical literature represents a selective and biased subset of study outcomes[72] and often promotes new drugs that have no greater benefit than existing treatments.

Meta-Analysis

Meta-analysis is a technique that is increasingly used to summarize results from a number of clinical trials. One recent analysis suggested that antioxidant vitamins increase the risk of death.[73] However, the researchers selected a small number (68) of papers from the many (16,111) they initially considered. The selection was carried out by the researchers themselves with full knowledge of the results of the studies. Clearly, an unconscious bias on the part of the researchers could produce a misleading result.[74] Consistent with media predispositions against supplements, this paper was given a high profile, both in the general news and in medical reporting. Vitamin C provides a particular target for these inaccurate accounts, and the steady over-reporting of vitamin C scare stories is likely to contribute to the public's gradually eroding confidence in the medical establishment.

Conventional medicine's failure to even consider the effects of massive doses of vitamin C on a range of illnesses is a result of assuming that it has been "proven" that only low doses are needed. As we have seen, researchers erroneously suggested that the body was saturated at only 200 mg and no more would be absorbed. With this background, it is understandable that the apparently wild claims for larger doses of vitamin C were considered unscientific. After all, doctors may have thought, it is only vitamin C, a harmless white powder, found in fruit. Even if a vitamin tablet makes you feel better, they could attribute this to a placebo effect.

The problem is that the case against vitamin C is weak, and both the size of the doses and the claimed efficacy are much greater than conventional medicine could apparently comprehend. Placebo-controlled clinical trials are a "gold standard" in medicine but are often viewed with suspicion by the public and scientists from more rigorous disciplines. The claims for the efficacy of vitamin C are objective, uniquely large effects and cannot be explained as placebo. Reliance on clinical trials and "proof" holds back advances in medicine. All medical treatments depend for their justification on the basic sciences of biophysics, biochemistry, and physiology. Vitamin C has such justification.

CHAPTER 5

The Need for Antioxidants

*"The truth is, the science of Nature has been already too long
made only a work of the brain and the fancy. It is now high
time that it should return to the plainness and soundness
of observations on material and obvious things."*
—ROBERT HOOKE, *MICROGRAPHIA*

Scientists suggest that long ago, before life evolved, the earth's atmosphere contained little oxygen. However, as primitive microorganisms
and plants progressed, they developed the capacity to use energy from sunlight to make their own food (glucose) from water and carbon dioxide,
giving oxygen as a byproduct. This process is called photosynthesis and,
directly or indirectly, it provides the energy for most life on earth. Over
millions of years, the concentration of oxygen in the atmosphere grew
higher, allowing the evolution of organisms that use oxygen to burn fuels
to create the energy for life, as we do.

All life is based on chains of carbon, hydrogen, nitrogen, and oxygen
atoms, which bond together by sharing electrons to form molecules.
Unfortunately, oxygen has a penchant for a somewhat one-sided sharing.
Oxygen's strong electron pull distorts such organic molecules by stealing
some of their electrons, a process known as oxidation. In an increasingly
oxygen-rich atmosphere, organic molecules would combine with oxygen
and their structure would be damaged.

A spectacular example of the process of oxidation familiar to us all is
burning. For example, when we burn coal for heat or petroleum in car
engines, the coal or gas is oxidized. The process does not have to be so
dramatic, however. If cooking oil is exposed to the air, it deteriorates slow-

ly, combining with oxygen. The same is true when a cut apple turns brown. This reaction requires energy, but is essentially similar to slow burning. The energy supply for our bodies also involves oxidation: we slowly metabolize or "burn" molecules from our food, producing chemical energy. As a result, every cell in our body needs a constant supply of oxygen to feed our internal biochemical fires. Antioxidants, such as vitamin C, are substances that help prevent damage to the body from oxygen.

Oxidation and Free Radicals

A cell is the smallest unit of life: it can maintain itself, grow, and reproduce. Most organisms, such as bacteria, exist as single-celled creatures, able to thrive without much cooperation with others. To create larger organisms, cells need to cooperate. Single-celled organisms do not have arms, legs, or eyes, thus have a limited scope for interacting with their environments. Large multicellular animals have the advantages of sight, organized movement, and thought, as a result of cooperation between cells. Living cells need oxygen to burn food and produce energy. The main exception to this rule is anaerobic bacteria, which cannot live in the presence of oxygen. However, most cells have evolved antioxidant defenses to provide essential barriers to the poisonous effects of too much oxidation.

Oxygen has the paradoxical property that, although it is essential to life, it can also be a deadly poison. We need oxygen to metabolize food, but it can also attack our own body tissues. One reason may be that our tissues are similar to the food we eat, since they are made of the same molecules: the building blocks of our bodies and cells are organic molecules consisting largely of water, proteins, and fats. Both meat and vegetables in our food are composed of these same materials.

To prevent such damage, our cells have evolved numerous antioxidants. An antioxidant is the name given to any mechanism or substance that prevents oxidation. Our cells use a substantial proportion of their energy to manufacture a large array of antioxidants, which shows how important these mechanisms are. Biological cells are full of antioxidants, which protect them from the oxidizing environment, but this protection takes energy. Thus, a sliced apple exposed to air turns brown, as its antioxidant defenses are overwhelmed by exposure to oxygen. Most diseases and features of aging also involve oxidation reactions.

Pure oxygen can kill cells and tissues, but the damaging process of oxidation does not require oxygen—many other molecules share this chemical property. Any substance that can steal electrons from other molecules is called an oxidant. For example, ultraviolet light and x-rays can knock electrons out of organic molecules, causing oxidation. Such ionizing radiation creates free radicals.

Free radicals are energetic molecules that can cause oxidation and tissue damage. Before we can understand what a free radical is, we must look more closely at the structure of atoms and molecules. Atoms contain a nucleus of neutrons and protons surrounded by a cloud of electrons. An electron has a negative electrical charge that generates a magnetic field as it spins. In molecules, most electrons exist in stable pairs, each spinning in opposite directions so that their magnetic fields cancel each other out.

A free radical is a reactive molecule with one or more unpaired electrons, which can be highly reactive.[1] This means trouble, because these energetic molecules will grab electrons from other molecules. Since atoms and molecules in the body are constantly vibrating and moving about, free radicals can rip electrons right out of essential proteins or even DNA. Uncontrolled free radical reactions cause tissue damage too. What is worse, free radicals can produce chain reactions within our cells, as one molecule after another becomes oxidized.

Oxygen, as you might expect, is a free radical. The unique chemistry of oxygen is partly a result of it being stable despite having two unpaired electrons. It has two electrons spinning in the same direction, which makes it magnetic. Magnetic substances, like iron, have at least one unpaired electron. The phrase "reactive oxygen species" describes a number of free radicals and energetic molecules derived from oxygen. Some reactive oxygen species are not free radicals but rather highly energetic oxidants. These produce free radicals within tissues and include hydrogen peroxide, hypochlorous acid, ozone, and singlet (one-atom) oxygen. Reactive species can also be formed from nitrogen and from chlorine, as found in common household bleach.

Types of Free Radicals

Superoxide molecule is a reactive oxygen species. It is similar to the oxygen molecule (O_2), but the superoxide molecule is oxygen packing an additional electron ($\cdot O_2^-$). It does not live up to its dazzling name, however, as it is not very reactive. While superoxide reacts rapidly with free radicals, its reactions with organic molecules in the cell require an acidic environment.

The most abundant substance in our bodies is water. Water molecules consist of two atoms of hydrogen and one of oxygen (H_2O). Several important free radicals are related to this simple molecule. The hydroxyl ion ($\cdot OH$) is water that has lost a hydrogen atom. The dot ($\cdot$) in the formula indicates that it has an unpaired electron. Hydroxyl ions are highly energetic and particularly damaging: they react instantaneously with almost any molecule they meet on their rapid diffusion through a cell. Without a large concentration of antioxidants, a hydroxyl radical can trigger a chain of damaging reactions.

If a hydroxyl ion steals an electron from an essential protein or DNA molecule, it becomes inert or unreactive. However, the molecule it stole the electron from now has an unpaired electron and has itself become a free radical. This sequence is called a free radical chain reaction. This chemical chain letter continues until one of the molecules changes its essential structure, disabling its function. Alternatively, it may be stopped by an antioxidant donating an electron to render the free radical safe and stop the damaging chain of events.

Addition of an oxygen atom to water forms hydrogen peroxide (H_2O_2). Hydrogen peroxide is well known for its action as an oxidizing agent in hair bleach, but in much higher concentration it can be used as rocket fuel. This potentially reactive molecule is present within our cells and tissues, fortunately at a low level. While hydrogen peroxide is normally considered harmful, recent research suggests that it is an essential part of signaling mechanisms used for cellular control. Higher concentrations of hydrogen peroxide act as an oxidizing agent, especially in the presence of iron or copper. This reaction with iron produces destructive hydroxyl radicals and free radical damage. The reaction of hydrogen peroxide with iron is given the name "the Fenton reaction" in general chemistry, named after the chemist Henry Fenton, who described the reaction at the end of the nineteenth century.

Antioxidants and Reduction

Antioxidants prevent oxidation damage by donating electrons to replace those lost to oxidation. This process of providing electrons is the reverse of oxidation and is called reduction.

Antioxidants are called free radical scavengers because they neutralize free radicals in the body. An antioxidant, such as vitamin C, can donate electrons to the free radical, thus stopping the free radical from stealing another electron. Vitamin C's donated electron allows the maverick free radical electron to form a balanced pair.

Oxidation: losing an electron

Reduction: gaining an electron

In the example of a cut apple, we can prevent the browning by applying an antioxidant. If the apple is left untreated, oxygen in the air oxidizes the surface tissue, pulling out electrons and turning it brown almost immediately. A solution of vitamin C, or lemon juice, applied to the cut surface of the apple slows down the oxidation process. The surface of a treated apple will stay fresh and white for a considerable time. The addition of vitamin C provides a supply of antioxidant electrons, preventing damage and discoloration. Antioxidants are often added to food, such as deli meats or bread, to maintain shelf life and freshness.

The apple experiment illustrates something more profound than the simple preservation of food. It shows how a living tissue can be damaged by oxidation and, more importantly, how an antioxidant can maintain tissue health. The uncut apple sealed within its skin is sheltered from the air and oxidation damage; its natural antioxidants can maintain the health of the unexposed tissue. When exposed, however, its antioxidants are insufficient to prevent the damage. The cut apple may be protected from oxidation by addition of an antioxidant. Similarly, our tissues have adequate antioxidant defenses to provide for a lifespan of about eighty years. However, these defenses are insufficient to prevent the damaging oxidation reactions in acute illness or chronic disease.

Our tissues maintain a controlled balance of reduction and oxidation, called the "redox state." Cells produce antioxidants and antioxidant electrons continuously in order to prevent oxidation damage. When the supply of energy from metabolism is disturbed, the balance between oxidants and antioxidants breaks down. An example of this is the damage caused by heart attacks or occlusive strokes. In these conditions, an artery supplying the tissue is blocked by a blood clot, leaving the tissue deprived of oxygen. The cells are unable to generate sufficient metabolic energy, so they divert energy away from production of antioxidant electrons. If the artery opens again (for example, if the blood clot dissolves), oxygen rushes into the tissue and the cells find themselves right back in an oxi-dizing redox environment, but now with a shortage of antioxidants. As a result, heart or brain tissues that survived the original insult may die. The now abundant supply of oxygen triggers a massive burst of free radicals that kills and damages cells. This process is described as reperfusion dam-age and it may be inhibited by supplying suitable antioxidants.[2]

The Body's Premier Water-Soluble Antioxidant

Oxidation and reduction are essential to life. Too high a concentration of oxygen poisons tissues, producing free radical damage, which can be pre-vented by antioxidants. Vitamin C is the most important water-soluble antioxidant in our diet. It is also the main water-soluble antioxidant in plants and is essential for growth.[3] Its great abundance in plant tissue allows us to prevent acute scurvy by eating a relatively small amount of fruits and vegetables. Its synthesis in large amounts in both plants and most animals suggests that higher levels may be essential for good health.

Vitamin C is unusual in that it has two antioxidant electrons that it can donate to prevent oxidation. When ascorbic acid donates one electron, it becomes the ascorbyl radical, which is relatively unreactive, short-lived, and harmless. This lack of reactivity enables vitamin C to intercept dan-gerous free radicals, donating an electron to satisfy their demand, and thus preventing damage. If an ascorbyl radical donates its second electron, it forms dehydroascorbate. Dehydroascorbate is an oxidized form and can be reduced (given electrons) back to ascorbate, the vitamin C molecule. This reduction and replenishment of vitamin C is performed within cells, but it requires electrons from the cellular metabolism. The metabolic processes in a cell serve two main purposes—to provide chemical energy for reactions and to generate high-energy antioxidant electrons to main-tain the redox state of the cell. High doses of vitamin C are unique in that they can provide the cell with a supply of antioxidant electrons without drawing on the cell's essential energy supply. This is useful for healthy cells, but damaged and stressed cells gain a double benefit—a supply of antioxidant electrons and an energy boost.

In Sickness and In Health

Oxidation and free radicals cause disease. Healthy tissue has high levels of ascorbate and low levels of its oxidized form, dehydroascorbate. In the oxidizing environment of sick tissues, vitamin C protects the cells from damage, becoming oxidized to dehydroascorbate in the process.[4] An increase in oxidized vitamin C has been shown in many different conditions. Tissue damage in surgery can increase the level of dehydroascorbate relative to ascorbate.[5] Diabetics have increased oxidative stress and higher dehydroascorbate levels.[6] High levels of oxygen increase dehydroascorbate in mice.[7] Similarly, mice with inflammation and arthritis have higher levels of dehydroascorbate. Diabetic kidneys increase vitamin C oxidation in rats, as does inflammation, but antioxidant supplementation can inhibit this effect.[8] Other free radical scavengers, such as glutathione, the most abundant antioxidant in cells, can also be used as indicators of damage or poor health.[9] The proportion of oxidized glutathione is a measure of tissue damage. Vitamin C and glutathione work together to maintain tissue health.[10]

Most animals manufacture vitamin C internally and increase production when sick, thus increasing their ascorbate to dehydroascorbate ratio. This helps return the sick tissues to a healthy, reduced state. Humans, however, having lost the ability to make vitamin C internally, compensate by increasing absorption from the gut: *when sick, humans can absorb far more dietary vitamin C,* which may help them through the crisis. This response of increasing absorption will only work if there is an abundance of vitamin C in the diet. Since modern human diets generally have a low vitamin C content, the increased absorption will be ineffective unless the person is using dietary supplements.

Earlier, we saw that applying a vitamin C solution to a cut apple prevents browning and oxidation, at least for a short time. Ultimately, however, the electrons provided by the added vitamin C will be used up and the surface of the apple will eventually turn brown. When the vitamin C has been oxidized, it can no longer protect the apple's surface. Many dietary antioxidants provide a similarly limited resistance to oxidation. If an antioxidant, such as vitamin E, enters an inflamed or damaged tissue, it will donate electrons to prevent some of the free radical damage. Having donated its electrons, it becomes unable to continue its function as an antioxidant. However, in healthy tissues, metabolism provides energy and electrons to regenerate antioxidants.

Vitamins C and E can act to transfer these antioxidant electrons to free radicals before they can cause damage. Unfortunately, in damaged or sick tissues, cells are under stress and may be unable to provide enough antioxidant electrons from their stressed energy supply to prevent further oxidation damage. Under these conditions, vitamins C and E are described as being rate-limited, since they can only donate electrons at the speed at which they are provided by the cell's metabolism. Fortunately, as Robert F. Cathcart III suggested, vitamin C is a nontoxic, non-rate-limited antioxidant available in the diet.[11]

Suppose, instead of painting the surface of the apple, we allowed a solution of vitamin C to continuously flow across it. The apple could then be maintained in its white, pristine condition, protected by the flow of vitamin C and antioxidant electrons. As the vitamin C molecules donate their electrons, other molecules immediately replace them and the electron supply would be maintained in abundance. Given a constant flow of vitamin C, even a sick or damaged tissue could remain in a reduced (non-oxidized) state.

Vitamin C is different from the other dietary antioxidants, such as vitamin E or selenium. Other antioxidants do not have the properties needed for vitamin C's unique antioxidant effect. Some, like selenium, are more toxic and cannot be given in massive doses. Coenzyme Q_{10} is nontoxic but more fat-soluble and thus is retained in the body, unable to provide the necessary flow. Vitamin E, a mixture of tocopherols and tocotrienol molecules, is also fat-soluble and a large molecule. Ascorbic acid is a small, water-soluble molecule with an exceedingly low toxicity, so it can be given in massive doses (up to 200 grams a day) to provide large amounts of free antioxidant electrons. Dr. Cathcart, who used massive doses to treat disease, first described the potential for vitamin C to act in this way and more recently helped extend this approach to the dynamic flow model.[12] In dynamic flow, the body is maintained in a reducing state, in health or disease, by a continuous large intake of vitamin C.

The body can absorb a sustained large intake of vitamin C, which is distributed around the body. However, at the same time it is being absorbed into the body, the kidneys are rapidly removing vitamin C from the blood. Just like in the flow across the cut apple, the body can now be maintained in a reduced state with minimal free radical damage. Oxidized vitamin C no longer needs to be regenerated by energy from metabolism; it is simply excreted and replaced by fresh intake. A sick cell is in an oxidized state and needs a constant supply of antioxidant electrons and energy. By supplying free antioxidant electrons, dynamic flow vitamin C saves the cell energy and protects it by providing abundant antioxidant electrons.

Vitamin C Therapy

Pharmacological doses of vitamin C, as are used to treat disease, should not be confused with basic nutrition. A person may take, for example, 8 grams (8,000 mg) a day to provide antioxidant protection and lower the incidence of infection, and such an intake would be effective *provided it was spread through the day in divided doses*. However, at the first sign of a cold, this relatively high nutritional intake would need to be dramatically increased.

People have been misled about the intakes needed for treating the common cold. Many people think the orthomolecular claim is that you should take a gram or two as a treatment. This is a myth. The actual recommendations for vitamin C in treatment of illness are larger. Typically, the dose is increased tenfold or more. The Vitamin C Foundation recommends taking at least 8 grams (8,000 mg) of vitamin C every twenty minutes for 3–4 hours until bowel tolerance, and then smaller dosages every 4–6 hours to prevent recurrence."[13] The apparently large 8-gram nutritional dose is now a minimum to be repeated every twenty minutes!

Dr. Cathcart has provided estimates of the amount of vitamin C needed to reach bowel tolerance (loose stool) in various diseases. These values range from around 30 grams (30,000 mg) for a mild cold to over 200 grams (200,000 mg) for viral pneumonia. *An individual's bowel tolerance level is proportional to the severity of their illness.* Many people have claimed that vitamin C does not work against the common cold; generally, these are people who take only a gram or two and expect a therapeutic response. *You need the amount of vitamin C that your body indicates it needs—not the amount you think you should take, but the amount that does the job.* Oddly enough, orthomolecular physicians and conventional doctors both agree on this: a gram of vitamin C is not an effective treatment for the common cold. The difference is that conventional doctors assume this means that vitamin C can be discounted, while the orthomolecular view is that a 1-gram dose is ridiculously small.

Conventional medicine's evident confusion over nutritional and pharmacological doses is not necessarily innocent. When Linus Pauling first published his book *Vitamin C and the Common Cold*, the establishment attacked him without sympathy or consideration of the science. Throughout his career, Dr. Pauling had been involved in scientific disputes, but this was something of a different nature. To try to brand one of the leading scientists of all time as a quack because he suggested that vitamin C could help against the common cold was odd. It seems strange that the medical establishment would get so upset over a simple vitamin and the common cold. Surely, some of the detractors had read the literature and were aware of the evidence for the effects of massive doses. Notably, if the claims for vitamin C were accepted, pharmaceutical companies might lose more than a few profits from cold medications.

If clinical studies with appropriate doses of vitamin C had been performed, there might be no vitamin C controversy. However, since Dr. Pauling's book, conventional medicine has been careful to avoid doing (and therefore having anyone read) studies on massive doses of vitamin C. By defining a single gram of vitamin C as a large dose, repeated clinical trials have studied limited doses in the range of up to a gram or so. These "high doses" of vitamin C, in the range of 500–1,500 mg, have repeatedly been shown to have a mixed and inconsistent effect on the progress of a common cold. Now you can see why that is so. The media is quick to notice these studies, preferentially disseminating negative information to the public and inaccurately assuring people that vitamin C is ineffective.

There is a huge difference between the size of the suggested therapeutic doses and those used merely to investigate vitamin C's nutritional properties. Therapeutic doses are more than 1,000 times the Recommended Dietary Allowance (RDA)/Dietary Reference Intake (DRI) value. Comparing the nutritional doses to pharmacological doses of vitamin C is equivalent to suggesting a small tree is similar in height to Mount Everest: just as no one would suggest a child requires oxygen or an ice axe to climb a tree, orthomolecular doctors do not claim that gram-level doses of vitamin C will cure disease.

One of the first scientists to realize that massive doses of vitamin C could force the body into a reducing state, and thus help combat disease, was Irwin Stone, Ph.D. He noticed that a range of diseases increase the ratio of oxidized to reduced vitamin C: the more severe the illness, the greater the oxidation.[14] Over time, this led to the idea that perhaps a disease process requires oxidation and produces an excess of free radicals. If this is the case, then a dynamic flow of vitamin C might neutralize free radicals, returning sick tissue to a reducing redox state. Vitamin C modifies cell signaling, modulates the body's immune response, prevents shock, and lowers inflammation. The body's response to stress is optimal in a reducing environment. If correct, this would mean that vitamin C could protect against a wide range of insults and disease states.

Frederick R. Klenner, M.D., suggested that, in human disease, vitamin C follows the law of mass action: in reversible reactions, the extent of chemical change is proportional to the active masses of the interacting substances. In other words, the more vitamin C taken, the greater is the effect. Giving low megadoses might, at best, suppress symptoms while prolonging the duration of the disease. In the intervening half century, other physicians such as Drs. Robert Cathcart, Abram Hoffer, and Tom Levy have repeatedly reported similar observations. These clinical observations are consistent with all the known scientific facts and, given the size of the reported effects, cannot be explained by the placebo effect.

The aim of vitamin C therapy is to keep the ratio of ascorbate to dehydroascorbate high. This is accomplished by keeping the incoming supply on the high side. Doing so will provide damaged cells with a reducing environment and will facilitate their recovery. Typically, antioxidants are engaged in a continuous oxidation-reduction cycle, and this cycling uses energy from the metabolic pathways of the cell.[15] Remember that stressed cells are unable to regenerate sufficient antioxidants to meet the increased demand, and that's why we have to come to their rescue with high doses of ascorbate.

Our tabletop model for this damage and stress is a cut apple. By supplying sufficient vitamin C in a continuous flow, we can keep the apple's surface in a pristine state. This process can work with other tissues. Massive doses of vitamin C will extinguish most free radicals and replenish antioxidants that have become oxidized. It enhances redox signaling within the damaged tissue, helping to provide an appropriate healing response to the illness.

The flow of fresh vitamin C through the body means that diseased cells get a large "free" supply of antioxidant electrons, lowering the demand on the cells' energy metabolism. Massive doses of vitamin C free other molecules from acting as antioxidants and help restore normal metabolic function.[16] Vitamin C provides injured cells with a free supply of antioxidant electrons, helping return the injured body to good health.

The body's need for vitamin C increases dramatically when sick. The amount of vitamin C a person can absorb increases as health decreases. Providing a dynamic flow of vitamin C through the body returns the damaged tissue back to a reducing state and health.

CHAPTER 6

Infectious Diseases

"Do not let yourself be tainted with a barren skepticism."
—LOUIS PASTEUR (ATTRIBUTED)

A reader of the DoctorYourself.com website relayed a story about how, one Monday morning some years ago, he had a fever of 102°F, although normally he rarely suffered illness. He immediately set about taking 10 grams (10,000 mg) of vitamin C *each hour,* expecting to get loose stools quickly. However, despite this massive intake, he did not reach bowel tolerance on the first day. The next day, he increased the dose to 15 grams each hour. Two days later, still feeling sick, he endeavored to take an entire bottle of vitamin C (250 grams). He would have arranged an intravenous infusion, but he was unwell and no doctors nearby provided this therapy. He gradually became annoyed by the fact that he could not induce loose stools. On Friday, a friend took him to a local hospital to ensure that he was not seriously ill. The hospital recommended that he be admitted but were unable to provide an immediate diagnosis. He declined the offer and went home, where he continued taking massive amounts of vitamin C. On Saturday night, his fever broke, with profuse sweating. He went to an internist, who declared him to be in perfect health.

Two weeks earlier, this same man had received emergency calls from the health department. Three people from a hotel where he had stayed had become ill with similar symptoms. Each had gone to a different hospital and had died, a few days later, from Legionnaires' disease, a rare form of pneumonia that may follow inhalation of minute droplets of water contaminated with *Legionella* bacteria.[1] Severe Legionnaires' disease has an overall mortality rate of 10–30 percent,[2] and 30–50 percent of patients need intensive care.[3] Following blood tests, one of the nation's leading Legionnaires' disease experts confirmed that the man had a fatal form of legionellosis. The physician initially doubted the validity of the results, which were confirmed by a second test. The doctor seemed surprised that the subject had survived . . . and then stated that vitamin C could not be a factor. Some medical practitioners persist in the rather unscientific denial of the effectiveness of vitamin C in such conditions; in this case, the physician had no direct evidence upon which to base such a statement. The patient, however, now had a satisfactory explanation for not achieving bowel tolerance, even with huge oral intakes of vitamin C.

Pneumonia

The anecdote about vitamin C's action in Legionnaires' disease is intriguing, but vitamin C is also reported to be an effective treatment for more common forms of pneumonia. Here, we use pneumonia to represent the large number of infectious diseases for which people have claimed vitamin C to be an effective treatment or even cure.[4]

Prevention is obviously easier than treating severe illness. Immediate use of hourly gram doses of vitamin C up to saturation will usually stop bronchitis or pneumonia from ever starting. Robert F. Cathcart III, M.D., advocated treating pneumonia with up to 200,000 mg (200 grams) of vitamin C daily, often taken intravenously. (Pneumonia is a severe disease and needs immediate medical attention by a qualified physician. Also, intravenous sodium ascorbate should only be administered by a doctor.) A person can simulate this process by taking vitamin C in frequent large doses by mouth. When one of the authors (A.W.S.) had pneumonia, he took 2,000 mg of vitamin C every six minutes to reach saturation. His daily dose was over 100,000 mg (100 grams). Fever, cough and other symptoms were reduced in hours and complete recovery took just a few days. This response was comparable to that expected from an antibiotic, but the ascorbate was both safer and cheaper.

The early vitamin C pioneers treated respiratory and other infections with massive amounts of vitamin C, so this is not a new idea at all. Both Frederick R. Klenner, M.D., and William McCormick, M.D., used this approach successfully for decades beginning in the 1940s! Clinical reports have repeatedly confirmed the powerful antibiotic-antiviral effect of vitamin C when used in sufficient quantity.

Vitamin C can be used alone or along with conventional medications, if one so chooses. However, currently, prescription drugs and conventional treatment leave a lot to be desired, as each year 75,000 Americans die from pneumonia.[5] Conventional medicine has never tried massive doses of vitamin C for this or other infections, and considering the positive clinical reports and the annual cost in lives, there is no excuse for excluding it.

AIDS and Other Viral Diseases

Vitamin C in sufficient doses has been claimed to be the most effective treatment of viral infections from the common cold to polio. An especially powerful example is provided by the early work on acquired immunodeficiency syndrome (AIDS). As might be expected, Dr. Cathcart was the first physician to report that full-blown AIDS could largely be reversed with a sufficient intake of vitamin C.[6] He reported on a group of approximately ninety AIDS patients who took high doses of vitamin C independently; an additional twelve of his AIDS patients were described, six of whom received intravenous ascorbate. Dr. Cathcart reported a response proportionate to the amount of vitamin C consumed. Only one patient had died, and he had previously received whole-body irradiation and chemotherapy (presumably for cancer), plus intravenous ascorbate could not be administered as the patient's veins had been so damaged by prior therapy. Australian physician Professor Ian Brighthope replicated Dr. Cathcart's work. In 1987, he published *The AIDS Fighters*, in which he reported, "We have to date not had a single death amongst our patients with full-blown AIDS who have continued on our vitamin C and nutrition program."[7]

Vitamin C was not considered by conventional medicine as a treatment for AIDS even before anti-retroviral drugs were available. There were no clinical trials, and physician reports were ignored or sidelined. Twenty years later, the suggestion for the use of vitamin C has become politically controversial. In Africa, where the population cannot afford the conventional patented drug therapies, the use of vitamin C–based treatments is attacked without providing clinical evidence in support.[8] "In an unprecedented action, the World Health Organization (WHO), the United Nations (UNICEF), and an AIDS activist group that promotes drug therapy in South Africa, joined forces in opposing vitamin therapy that exceeds the Recommended Dietary Allowance (RDA), and in particular vitamin C in doses they describe as being 'far beyond safe levels'."[9]

Dr. Cathcart proposed trying vitamin C therapy on emerging viral diseases such as the deadly Ebola virus, for which there is no effective treatment. Ebola hemorrhagic fever has a 60–80 percent mortality rate, so if you get the disease the odds are that you will die from it. Dr. Cathcart argued that Ebola and its relatives induce an acute scurvy and intravenous ascorbate should be tried in these patients. He noted that the first subject who recovered from another emerging disease—Lassa fever, another viral hemorrhagic fever—had been taking vitamins.[10] Dr. Cathcart suggested that intravenous doses of perhaps 500 grams of sodium ascorbate would be required. Despite having no effective treatment, conventional medicine to date has not tried massive infusions of sodium ascorbate, which may provide the only effective treatment currently available.

Quantity, Frequency, and Duration

A therapeutic level of vitamin C supplementation used by Dr. Klenner is 350 mg of vitamin C per kilogram (1 kg = approximately 2.2 pounds) of body weight per day.[11] The following table provides a working summary:

THERAPEUTIC LEVELS OF VITAMIN C SUPPLEMENTATION			
BODY WEIGHT	VITAMIN C PER DAY	NUMBER OF DOSES	INDIVIDUAL DOSE
100 kg (220 lbs)	35,000 mg	17–18	2,000 mg
75 kg (165 lbs)	26,000 mg	17–18	1,500 mg
50 kg (110 lbs)	18,000 mg	18	1,000 mg
25 kg (55 lbs)	9,000 mg	18	500 mg
12.75 kg (28 lbs)	4,500 mg	9	500 mg.
7 kg (15.5 lbs)	2,300 mg	9	250 mg
3.5 kg (7.5 lbs)	1,200 mg	9	130–135 mg

In orthomolecular medicine, these are moderate oral doses. Dr. Klenner actually used as much as four times this amount, typically by injection of sodium ascorbate. He recommended daily preventive doses for the healthy, which might be about a fifth of the above therapeutic amounts, divided into four doses daily.

At a sufficient intake, vitamin C has antihistamine, antitoxin, antibiotic, and antiviral properties. Its nature and safety does not change with the dose, but its power and effectiveness does. If it takes about fifty gallons of gas to drive from New York City to Albuquerque, you simply are not going to make it on ten gallons, no matter how you try. Likewise, if your body wants 35,000 mg of vitamin C to fight an infection, 7,000 mg won't do. The key is to take enough C, take it often enough, and take it long enough.

Quantity, frequency, and duration are the keys to effective orthomolecular use of vitamin C in infections. Many people hold a philosophical viewpoint that "I shouldn't have to take so much of a vitamin." It's certainly true that you do not have to—everyone has the right to be sick if they want to. However, if you want the possibility of a swift recovery, and if you want to use vitamin C, you should use it effectively: frequent doses up to bowel tolerance. Rather than take what we think the body should require, we should take the amount of C that the body says it wants.

It is important to remember that experienced physicians such as Dr. Cathcart have used daily doses of 200,000 mg with safety. The major side effect of vitamin C overload is an unmistakable diarrhea. This indicates absolute saturation, and the daily dose is then dropped to the highest amount that will not bring about diarrhea. That intake is often a therapeutic level.

Clinical Success

In 1975, Dr. Cathcart reported that, over a three-year period, he had treated more than 2,000 patients with massive doses of vitamin C.[12] He noted considerable beneficial effects in acute viral disease and suggested that a clinical trial would substantiate his observations. Regrettably, clinical trials of these large doses have not been performed. In 1981, he documented a further 7,000 patients who had been given the treatment, which had markedly altered the expected course of a large number of diseases.[13] Since that time, he has continued treating many thousands of patients, with similar positive results.

Dr. Cathcart reports surprisingly few problems with the massive doses he has tried, stating that the majority of patients have little difficulty with them. This is confirmed by the experience of other physicians giving high-dose ascorbate treatment.[14] Minor complaints, such as gas, diarrhea, or stomach acid, reported by some healthy people taking large oral doses of vitamin C, are rare in sick patients.

Below bowel tolerance levels, vitamin C generally has little effect on a disease process, whereas doses that are close to the bowel tolerance level can greatly reduce symptoms. Dr. Cathcart describes the effect of vitamin C at these doses as being clinically dramatic, as if a threshold had been reached.[15] His patients experienced a feeling of well-being at high dose levels and considered this an unexpected benefit. These feelings of well-being suggest no obvious detrimental side effect is present. Dr. Cathcart reports that in severe disease, such as viral pneumonia, the benefit is substantial; he describes a complete cessation of symptoms. Such a powerful effect is difficult to dismiss, either as a placebo response or as self-delusion on the part of the physician.

Importantly, in terms of relating the response to a dose of vitamin C, symptoms can be turned on or off by adjusting the dose. The sickness and acute symptoms of diseases such as pneumonia were found to return if the vitamin C levels were lowered. This process of switching symptoms on and off with the vitamin C dose is an important observation, since it means that the patients are acting as their own experimental controls. The authors have tried this experiment with the common cold and found that massive doses of ascorbate often bring substantial symptomatic relief and alleviate the "washed-out" feeling that accompanies a cold.

Titration to bowel tolerance levels is fine for people who can be persuaded to take huge amounts of vitamin C. However, if the disease is more severe, or the patient is unable to take large doses orally, then intravenous infusion of sodium ascorbate may be substituted. With intravenous ascorbate, the clinical effect is reported to be even more dramatic.

Other physicians and researchers working with massive doses of vitamin C report findings entirely consistent with those of Dr. Cathcart. Clinical reports of the beneficial action of these doses are often striking and patients with severe disease can recover rapidly. Australian physician Archie Kalokerinos has described seeing children in severe shock, unresponsive to treatment and on the point of death, recovering in a matter of minutes.[16] Either the medical establishment has overlooked an important finding or multiple independent physicians are each separately reporting a substantial effect that is specific to this vitamin and strangely is not obtainable with any other substance.

Throughout recent decades, doctors have independently been reporting astounding responses to the use of high doses of vitamin C in infectious disease. The doses employed have been about 100 times those used in conventional medicine and the medical establishment has never tested these claims scientifically.

CHAPTER 7

Cancer and Vitamin C

*"Growth for the sake of growth
is the ideology of the cancer cell."*
—EDWARD ABBEY

For most people, a diagnosis of cancer is a devastating experience, as it is one of the most feared diseases in the world. As average lifespan has increased, so has the incidence of this disease: one in three people will likely suffer from it, usually in their later years. It is therefore important to understand how and why cancer develops, and what we can do about it.

The fundamental role of vitamin C and other antioxidants in the prevention and control of this disease has only recently become clear. Reduction and oxidation (redox) chemicals signal cells to divide, to change their structure and behavior, or to die. One of the most critical controlling factors is the availability of vitamin C. High doses of vitamin C, in combination with related nutrients, may prevent or even cure cancer.

A Consequence of Evolution

In order to appreciate the role of vitamin C, we need to understand the mechanisms leading to cancer. Cancer is a disease of cells—a cancer forms when some cells stop cooperating with the rest of the body and begin acting as independent agents. Cells run amok in this way because of factors related to the way animals and plants have evolved over millions of years. For this reason, we can consider cancer, like aging, to be a consequence of evolution.

Biological evolution concerns changes in the inherited traits of living organisms over generations, resulting in the development of new species.

In evolutionary terms, humans are extremely recent: they began to emerge about 3 million years ago. Most of life's long history has been taken up with the evolution of single-celled microorganisms. Scientists have found traces of microbes in rocks that are 3.5 billion years old, whereas fossils of multicelled organisms are found only in rocks less than a billion years old.

Around 3 billion years ago, early cells developed the ability to photosynthesize, using energy from sunlight to create sugar from carbon dioxide and water, producing oxygen as a waste product. Directly or indirectly, nearly all life depends on this redox reaction. Redox reactions drive the chemistry of living organisms. In the early stages of evolution, vitamin C became the most abundant water-soluble antioxidant in plants, and animals also require vitamin C, often in large amounts. One reason for this need is that vitamin C is a central part of the controls that developed to prevent cancer in multicellular creatures such as humans.

Microorganisms and Multicellularity

For most of the history of life on Earth, living organisms consisted of single cells. Biologists classify these into groups that include bacteria, fungi, Archaea, and protists. Multicellular organisms took a long time to evolve, partly because of the increased levels of organization and cooperation they need. Keep in mind that single-celled organisms are not inferior to large, multicellular creatures; in many respects, they are biologically more successful. Single-celled organisms dominate the earth—they are the simplest, most diverse, and most widespread group of living organisms.

People are typically unaware of these microorganisms unless they are pathogenic. Pathogenic microbes are a leading cause of death and disease. Despite this harm, the continued existence of humans, plants, and animals on the Earth ultimately depends on the activities of numerous bacteria and other microorganisms. Surprisingly, many microorganisms are more effective chemical factories than animals and can exist on a few simple chemicals. These organisms have little need for exogenously supplied vitamin C.

Generally, single-celled organisms act independently, as their name suggests, although many produce colonies, which are not true multicellular organisms but a collection of single cells with minimal cooperation. Other primitive single-celled creatures, such as slime molds, band together when stressed, cooperating to produce a mobile fruiting body ("slug") in order to disperse and invade other habitats. This is a higher level of cooperation and reflects the origins of multicellularity. Through evolution, single cells have managed to cooperate with others to make the transition to forming multicellular organisms. In each case, the final multicellular form provided a survival advantage. One of the reasons that single-celled organisms cooperate is to gain a greater information-processing capability, as cooperative cells often need to interact with a demanding environment.[1]

The formation of a multicellular structure involves control mechanisms, as even simple colonies have to be organized. For example, slime mold cells release chemicals into the environment that cause nearby cells to aggregate into the mobile slug.[2] A similar release of chemicals causes some populations of bacteria to alter their gene expression.[3] Once a colony has formed, it has to develop and maintain its internal structure. Multicelled organisms are complex: a human arm consists of bone, muscle, fat, blood vessels, and nerves, arranged in a three-dimensional anatomy. In order for the arm to move in a coordinated way, cells cooperate to generate movement based on electrochemical signals from the brain.

Large multicellular organisms depend on vitamin C and other antioxidants for control of their internal organization, a dependency that arose in part with the need to prevent cancer and associated disorders. To form a complicated multicellular organism, such as a mammal, individual cells need to be tightly controlled. The local balance of oxidants and antioxidants, like vitamin C, are central to this control mechanism.

Cell Suicide

The most demanding example of control is when, during development, cells are instructed to die, often by a local increase in oxidation. Our bodies are formed by organizing cell growth and cell death to produce three-dimensional structures. In addition, cells are instructed to switch on some genes and switch off others, converting cells into different types, such as muscle cells, fat cells, or nerve cells (a process called differentiation). A classic example of cell death during development is the growth of individual fingers and toes. At first, the hand is like a mitten, but then the cells between what are to become its fingers die. The cells are constrained to enter a suicide program called apoptosis. Unless individual cells committed suicide upon a suitable signal, the structure of our bodies could not be formed. Thus, odd though it seems, cell suicide is absolutely essential to multicellular life.

By contrast, single cells evolved to maintain their existence under any conditions—this is their fight for life. Suicide is not a useful activity for a single-celled organism. Wouldn't even defective bacteria cling to life and avoid suicide? Although this viewpoint seems obvious, surprisingly, a form of cell suicide does occur in bacteria, and is associated with bacteria that form colonies. Such colony-forming behavior may require a way to suppress aberrant cells in order to evolve successfully.[4] Some unicellular organisms form complex communities that have several of the properties of multicellular organisms. More generally, bacteria exist in ecological communities; the plaque that forms on teeth is an example of one type known as a biofilm. Bacteria in dental plaque gain protection within the biofilm and can be difficult to eradicate, even with the mechanical abrasion of a toothbrush.

The programmed death of individual damaged cells can be beneficial to a multicellular community. The "self-destruct" function might be seen as akin to intentionally flooding compartments in a burning ship in order to keep the vessel intact. Once again, a signal used to control this process is the local level of oxidation. In the body, cell suicide could limit the spread of a viral infection, for example. Similarly, in times of shortage, dying cells might donate their bodies as nutrients to neighboring cells. However, such altruistic behavior does not help the individual bacterium that commits suicide. To explain cell suicide in an evolutionary context, dying needs to carry a survival advantage.

In multicellular organisms, this paradox may be overcome. Complex multicellular organisms generally consist of cells containing the same genes. Under some circumstances, the death of an individual cell increases the probability that other cells with the same (or similar) genes will survive. For example, a litter of nine puppies has trouble nursing from eight teats, and the harsh rule of evolution is that the loss of one puppy can increase the survival likelihood of the other eight. The loss of a single copy of the genes can allow many more copies to survive. Multicellular organisms similarly protect the integrity of the whole by sacrificing individual cells, which they instruct to commit suicide when needed.

But what happens if the cell refuses the suicide instruction? Since a single cell might begin to act independently at any point, multicellular organisms have to make such defections costly. Multicellular organisms have a range of penalties for cells that defect; for instance, they may send a redox signal instructing the cell to die. Nevertheless, if these controls are lost, or damaged by a chronic shortage of vitamin C and other antioxidants, a cell might start to grow and divide, irrespective of the needs of the whole body—this is what we refer to as cancer.

Are There Many Types of Cancer?

Physicians often describe cancer as a large number of different conditions, each involving abnormal cell division and growth. Cancers that arise in specific tissues, or with particular defining characteristics, are considered as individual diseases. The disadvantage of this approach is that it does not provide an overview of the biological mechanisms underlying the illness. However, the "many types" approach also has advantages, specifically in suggesting that some forms of cancer may be more susceptible to particular therapies. For example, hormone-based treatments may be more effective against cancers originating in hormonally responsive tissues, such as the prostate or breast, whereas a cancer originating in the lung might not respond favorably.

Clinically, cancer is often described in terms of the original site of the tumor. For example, "small cell lung cancer" is a type of cancer arising in the lung, which, as the name suggests, has relatively small cells. As cancer cells proliferate, they form tumors that may be benign or malignant. Many benign tumors are non-invasive and relatively safe, although some, such as uterine fibroids (which can occasionally lead to a hemorrhage or even death), may be life-threatening. Lumps of fatty tissue under the skin (lipomas) are a common form of a relatively harmless benign tumor.

Malignant tumors are the form of the disease that most people fear, and understandably so. A malignant tumor is an expanding mass of tissue that invades its surroundings, extending fingerlike into the tissues. The name *cancer* comes from the Greek word for "crab," as the invading protuberances were thought to resemble a crab's legs and claws. Malignant cancers do not have well-defined borders or a surrounding capsule. To the touch, a malignant tumor feels more attached to the neighboring tissues, in contrast to the clearly distinct lump that is characteristic of benign tumors.

Most tumors are classified into two main groups, carcinomas and sarcomas. Carcinomas originate from epithelial and endothelial tissues, which form the coverings of the external and internal surfaces of the body and include the skin and the linings of the mouth and gut. Carcinomas are common, because they arise in tissues that contain continuously dividing cells. Because of their protective function in the body, these tissues can be damaged by mechanical stress, chemical attack, or oxidation. Sarcomas are less common and derive from connective and non-epithelial tissues, such as bone, cartilage, muscle, or fat. Classifying malignant tumors into these different types is somewhat arbitrary, because cancers lose the characteristic features of the cells from which they arise.

The classification of cancers into particular types can be misleading and it obscures the similarities and the consistent changes in oxidation levels. The multiple disease approach also hides the central role of vitamin C in driving normal tissues into reducing states and sick tissues into oxidative states. Understanding the role of vitamin C and other antioxidants in the generation and growth of cancer brings us closer to the aim of cure.

A Single Disease

Viewing cancer as a single disease with many variants enables investigators to determine the core mechanisms. The primary feature of cancer is cell proliferation: a single cancer cell in a favorable environment, with an abundance of nutrients, can produce billions of offspring. A single aberrant cell can theoretically divide to form a large tumor. When growing rapidly, cancer cells may move and invade the surrounding tissues. During the infiltration of neighboring tissues, cancer cells overcome factors that normally limit tissue movement and growth. They often produce enzymes that break down the surrounding tissue matrix, enabling them to spread. This invasive process is both active and aggressive, and invasive tumors can even destroy bone.

Thinking of cancer as a single disease helps us to understand the process of carcinogenesis in terms of evolution. Cancer is the result of each individual cell's struggle to survive. We have seen that biology constructs multicellular organisms using a tight system of controls to enforce cellular cooperation and differentiation. However, these delicate controls developed in addition to earlier and tougher mechanisms that promote the survival of individual cells. Damaging a cell can break the continuity of these relatively fragile multicellular control mechanisms, leaving the earlier and more robust individual cell survival mechanisms. These mechanisms instruct the cell to survive by dividing, growing, and spreading—the fundamental characteristics of cancer.

In other words, cancer cells have the attributes of a biological organism that is struggling for survival in a hostile environment. By the time a cancer achieves malignancy, it is genetically different from the normal host cells. A typical cancer cell will have lost fragments of chromosomes and gained others. However, this idea is misleading, because there are no "typical" cells in malignant tumors. The cells differ widely, as errors in cell division have jumbled the chromosomes. One cancer cell might have only ten chromosomes, while another could have more than a hundred. A malignant cancer is actually an ecosystem containing competing single-celled organisms, each fighting to establish genetic success.

The simplest way of considering a malignant cancer cell is as a new species. Each cell is growing and trying to leave more offspring than its competitors. Cancer cells that grow rapidly, spread to new areas, and refuse to die will leave more offspring. By the laws of evolution, such "fitter" cells will survive. This is why cancer is so difficult to cure—cancer cells are successful survivors of an evolutionary battleground.

Multicellular organisms fight a constant battle with cancer. In order to survive, they have to prevent cancer from starting. If cancer does take hold, the healthy cells have a survival advantage if they can destroy it before it reduces their ability to survive. Thus, humans have evolved to resist cancer for long periods of their lives. Host resistance is often assumed to depend on the immune system to remove potentially cancerous cells. Redox substances provide an alternative and more general mechanism for removing aberrant cells, and an explanation for spontaneous remission.

Spontaneous remission with advanced cancers is rare, but it may involve the changes in the local redox state of the tissue. Over the years, hundreds of cases of spontaneous remission have been described.[5] Even by 1966, an estimated 200–300 accepted remissions had been recorded. However, unreported remissions may be much more numerous, as some people may remit before they have any symptoms and others may be on record as having been cured by the treatment they received when actually they recovered spontaneously. Local oxidation or destruction of tumors by the immune system could explain spontaneous remissions. A high intake of vitamin C will assist both the redox and immunological mechanisms behind spontaneous remissions. Indeed, one reason for the abundance of vitamin C and other antioxidants in both animals and plants is resistance to cancer.

Vitamin C and Cancer

In 1940, a few years after the vitamin C molecule was identified, researchers studied its effects in leukemia and noticed that cancer patients were often deficient in vitamin C.[6] It was thought that correcting this deficit with intravenous sodium ascorbate might be therapeutic. A little later, William J. McCormick, M.D., anticipated a relationship between cancer and shortage of vitamin C.[7] In his view, malignant cancer was a disease of inadequate collagen, resulting from a lack of vitamin C.

In 1969, it was shown that sufficiently high doses of vitamin C were actually toxic to malignant cancer cells. In the decade that followed, exciting research reports on vitamin C and cancer suggested a completely new approach to cancer prevention and treatment. Irwin Stone, Ph.D., also documented a relationship between a shortage of vitamin C and cancer.[8] He realized that vitamin C had produced a complete remission from leukemia in at least one report. A researcher had treated a patient suffering from myelogenous leukemia with 24–42 grams of vitamin C each day. The patient twice stopped taking the vitamin C and deteriorated, but when the vitamin C was reinstated, the illness went back into remission.[9]

This early research work led Drs. Linus Pauling and Ewan Cameron to perform their influential studies of vitamin C and cancer.[10] A number of Dr. Cameron's patients were cured.[11] Dr. Pauling reported that "the ascorbate-treated patients have lived, on the average, over five times as long as the matched control patients."[12] More recent research suggests that vitamin C–based redox mechanisms may be of great importance in protecting against carcinogenesis.[13] When an abnormal cell starts to divide, it becomes more oxidizing and may be more sensitive to redox and other signals to commit suicide by apoptosis.[14] The control mechanisms that multicellular organisms have evolved to combat the problem of cancer may provide new approaches to preventing and treating the disease.

Boosting Redox Mechanisms

Vitamin C is a unique antioxidant that keeps the body in a chemically reduced state. However, some scientists suggest that vitamin C can also act as an oxidant, and that oxidants cause damage to cells. They are factually correct, but far from this being a detriment to high doses, it may actually be useful in *protecting* us from cancer. Changes in the oxidation levels in cells are central to the development of cancer, but high levels of vitamin C can prevent these changes and inhibit carcinogenesis. Furthermore, in cancerous tissues, vitamin C acts as an oxidant, selectively killing the abnormal cells.

The redox state of a cell is an important biochemical property because the overall level of oxidation regulates genes and their expression. Cells use molecules, such as hydrogen peroxide, as signals both within and between cells. Oxidation and reduction control some of the more important aspects of cellular behavior, including the growth, multiplication, and death of cells. This control is a feature of all multicellular creatures and is one of the foremost mechanisms used to control cancer. The central role of vitamin C in the development and potential treatment of cancer arises from its dual roles as an antioxidant and an oxidant. Reduction and oxidation combine to control the mechanisms for cell division and death.

The overall redox state of cells is measured in millivolts (mV). Just as electricity involves a flow of electrons, the movement of electrons between molecules in bodily tissues produces a change in electric charge. Electrons carry a tiny negative charge. In a reducing environment with abundant antioxidants, more free electrons are available and the redox state (voltage) of the tissue is more negative. By contrast, a damaged tissue under free radical attack is in an oxidizing state and has fewer antioxidants. Oxidation and tissue damage is associated with a more positive redox state. Changes in the redox state are associated with different cellular behavior.[15] At rest, the redox state of the cell is relatively reducing, less than –260 mV, which corresponds to a healthy cell with an active antioxidant defense. Increased oxidation, perhaps signaled by a small increase in hydrogen peroxide or nitric oxide, increases the redox state to between –260 mV and –210 mV, leading to cell proliferation.

In general, cancer-causing agents induce oxidation or cell proliferation, which can increase any genetic errors that are present or have been caused by free radical damage. Rather than being a side effect of carcinogenesis, cell proliferation increases cell diversity and propels the cells toward malignancy. To prevent cancer developing, cells have inbuilt control mechanisms. As the redox state rises toward the oxidation level needed to produce overly rapid proliferation, cells attempt differentiation, which occurs between –210 mV and –180 mV. Cells that have changed into a more specialized form stop dividing. If a damaged cell cannot divide, it is unable to develop into a cancer—it may be sick or abnormal with little function, but it will not form a tumor.

A cell that refuses to differentiate faces another defense mechanism. As the redox level increases to between –180 mV and –160 mV, it triggers apoptosis, or programmed cell death. Since the host has been unable to save the cell by turning it into a specialized, non-dividing cell, it uses signals to instruct the cell to die. A dead cell can be cleared away efficiently, so it presents no particular threat to the host.

If a cell's apoptosis mechanism has been damaged and the cell refuses to commit suicide, there is a final mechanism available to protect the host. When the redox state becomes very oxidizing, above –150 mV, the cell dies immediately through necrosis. Whereas apoptosis restricts the release of cell contents and increased tissue damage, necrosis is catastrophic: the cell loses its structure and literally falls apart. The oxidation state has increased to the point where the cell is killed without due ceremony. Used as a high-dose treatment, vitamin C has been found to induce cancer necrosis in some patients.

Vitamin C and other antioxidants inhibit cell proliferation and the risk of cancer by maintaining an antioxidant redox state. The literature on tumor suppressor genes, such as *p53*, which actively prevent cancer, indicates that they act as antioxidants.[16] Conversely, genes that promote cancer (oncogenes) typically increase the oxidation state of the cell. Other cancer-causing and promoting agents, such as x-rays and ultraviolet radiation, also increase the redox state and cause free radical damage. An abundant supply of vitamin C provides free antioxidant electrons and may thus inhibit the development of cancer.[17]

A Nontoxic Anti-Cancer Agent

Vitamin C is a particularly useful anti-cancer agent because of its low toxicity. As we have explained, tumors are populations of cells that can evolve ways of resisting treatment, just as insects become resistant to pesticides or bacteria develop resistance to antibiotics. With treatments other than surgery, doctors hope to change the life/death balance so that more cancer cells die than are produced by cell division. If this is achieved, the tumor will shrink.

Oncologists use tumor shrinkage as a quantitative measure of the effectiveness of a therapy. Unfortunately, even if a treatment manages to shrink a tumor, it is not certain that the patient will live longer or suffer fewer symptoms. This poor result is because cells that are easy to kill are removed from the population, but the stronger cells that escape are highly resistant to the treatment, otherwise they would not have survived. The duration of conventional chemotherapy or radiation is usually relatively short, because it is poisonous to the patient's health, resulting in unbearable or even life-threatening side effects. If cancer cells remain following the treatment, the tumor can grow back with a higher proportion of resistant cells. The resistant cancer cells now face less competition for resources from other cancer cells, so they can often grow more rapidly. Subsequent treatments will be less effective, as the cells are less sensitive and selected for toughness. If the patient completes several cycles of treatment, the cancer cells can become completely resistant, and will then be free to grow and invade the body. Thus, the initial shrinking of a tumor is not a reliable indication of treatment success.

An effective therapy should increase the lifespan of the patients and increase their quality of life. It is important to consider the cost-benefit, pain-gain, relationship of conventional cancer therapies carefully for each patient. Typically, anti-cancer drugs are toxic chemicals that kill cells. In some cases, these toxic drugs kill cancer cells a little more effectively than they do healthy cells. When such drugs are given, the susceptible cells in the tumor may be wiped out quickly, but other susceptible cells, such as those in hair follicles and the lining of the gut, can also be damaged. With a sequence of treatments, cancer cells are selected for resistance, whereas the person's previously healthy cells become increasingly more damaged and unable to withstand the treatment.

The solution to this therapeutic impasse is to employ nontoxic anti-cancer agents. There are numerous such compounds available, but *the main component of an anti-cancer diet is vitamin C.* Vitamin C alone can be effective, but its action can be multiplied several-fold when combined with other redox nutrients and vitamins, such as alpha-lipoic acid or vitamin K_3. The nutrients act in redox-synergy to selectively destroy cancer cells. The driving force of this cancer destruction is the availability of massive amounts of vitamin C. A vitamin C–based approach can produce a constant pressure on the population of tumor cells, inhibiting their growth. But vitamin C acts as an antioxidant and protects healthy cells from the toxic effects of chemotherapy. In general, vitamin C does not appear to interfere with or reduce the effectiveness of chemotherapy.[18]

Vitamin C, acting as an oxidant, is selectively toxic to cancer cells, inhibiting their growth or killing them outright. Killing cancer using a redox-based nutritional approach has few side effects and there is evidence that it may increase lifespan, while enhancing the patient's quality of life. This is the good news about cancer and ascorbate.

A typical redox-synergy therapy based on vitamin C is given here.[19] This would be considered a standard approach for most cancer patients who are not in the final stages of the disease.

- Vitamin C (as L-ascorbic acid), dynamic flow level, at least 3 grams, five or six times each day, providing a daily total of 20 grams or more (>90 percent bowel tolerance). Liposomal formulations are highly recommended.

- R-alpha-lipoic acid, 200–500 mg with each dose of vitamin C (up to 5 grams total oral intake).

- Vitamin D_3, 4,000 IU per day.

- Selenium, 800 µG per day (as methylselenocysteine). This level of selenium intake corresponds to the U.S. government's "no observed adverse effect level" and is the maximum intake considered safe of any side effects.

- Absorbable magnesium, 400–2,500 mg per day (as magnesium citrate or magnesium chelate).

- Very-low-carbohydrate and low-calorie diet.

- Lots of fresh raw vegetables.

This is a severe dietary restriction, involving low calories and, in particular, reduced intake of carbohydrates and proteins. Essentially, it corresponds to severe dietary restriction with the highest tolerated intakes of vitamin C and alpha-lipoic acid.

Case Study

The following anecdote describes the experience of one of the authors (A.W.S) with a cancer patient taking large doses of vitamin C:

Joe had terminal lung cancer. He was constantly coughing up blood and

I talked with him in the living room of his small suburban home because Joe was too sick to come to my office. In fact, he was too sick to get out of his recliner. It was in this chair that his life was played out, day and night. He could not walk and he was in too much pain to even lie down. He spent the night in his chair. He did not want to eat. But he did still want to live, and he was willing to try even vitamins if they would help him feel any better.

It was October and the leaves, orange and bright yellow, were falling outside the picture window as we talked. It is never easy to work with the dying. As a counseling student, I'd seen plenty of them at the Brigham Hospital in Boston. Then, I had listened and watched—now, I listened and watched and suggested vitamin C.

"How much?" Joe croaked.

"As much as humanly possible under the circumstances," I replied. I explained bowel tolerance to him, and answered the usual questions from his family. Most centered on how well would it work. Some were understandably skeptical; some were in overly optimistic denial. "Vitamin C is very much worth using, with due consideration of how sick Joe really is." All agreed that Joe had nothing to lose.

Joe kept a big jug of water and a bottle of vitamin C crystals on the table right next to his recliner. Within days, Joe stopped coughing up the blood. This alone would have been more than enough benefit, but there was more good news within the week. His wife reported that Joe's appetite was back and he was able to lie down in bed. He was sleeping much better and in much less pain. Over and over, I have seen profound pain relief and dramatic improvement in sleeping in terminal patients that take huge doses of vitamin C. If the vitamin did nothing else, these benefits would be indisputable arguments for using it.

A week or so later, Joe was able to walk around the house with a cane and he was even walking around the yard. His wife was quite emotional as she reported his progress. She knew, at some level, that Joe was not likely to survive such severe cancer. And in the end, he didn't. But he added to his length of life, and the quality of that life was extraordinarily enhanced by the vitamin C.

How much did he take? About 4,000 mg every half hour when he was awake, day or night. That approaches 100,000 mg a day. Joe never got diarrhea. As time passes and our knowledge increases, we realize that the benefits of vitamin C for cancer patients can be greatly increased by its combination with other nutrients. Vitamin C works most effectively by driving a redox synergy with other nutrients, such as alpha-lipoic acid and vitamin K_3. Had this information been available at the time, Joe might have lived even longer and felt even better.

Cancer is one of the most feared diseases and its incidence and devastation has been increasing throughout modern history. The causes of this disease lie in the balance of oxidants and antioxidants in the cell. Humans are complex multicellular animals and have evolved numerous defenses against carcinogenesis and malignancy. A critical element in this defense is vitamin C.

CHAPTER 8

Heart Disease

"One sometimes finds what one is not looking for."
—ALEXANDER FLEMING

Vitamin C is critical for a healthy heart. People need not be dying from coronary heart disease or occlusive stroke because evidence suggests that an adequate intake of vitamin C and other antioxidants would prevent and potentially eliminate these conditions. Orthomolecular physicians have claimed for decades that the cause of heart attacks and strokes is low-grade scurvy. Ignoring this suggestion may have made these diseases the biggest killers in the Western world.

Strangely, however, deaths from these diseases were rare in the past—this is a new epidemic. It is not normally acknowledged that coronary heart disease is a relatively recent problem restricted to some humans living under modern conditions. Most animals do not suffer coronary heart attacks. Where it does occur in animals, it is rare and is associated with a lack of vitamin C. Something in the way people live has changed over the last hundred years or so, causing an epidemic of heart disease and stroke. These particular changes are not fully established or, more importantly, understood. The most that has been achieved is a statistical association with risk factors. However, there is a common clue—risk factors for heart disease directly or indirectly increase the body's need for vitamin C and other antioxidants.

The Heart and Circulation

In simple terms, the heart is the pump and the blood vessels are the piping used to transport blood about the body. The cardiovascular system has to be largely self-regulating and be able to repair itself quickly. It has many functions, but a single critical requirement is to deliver oxygen to the tissues.

Blood consists of cells in a surrounding fluid called plasma. Blood carries oxygen in red blood cells bound to a protein called hemoglobin. When bound to oxygen, hemoglobin is red, giving the blood its color. Red cells are the most abundant cells in the blood, consistent with their purpose in supplying the body with oxygen. When the blood supply to an organ is prevented, the tissues are deprived of oxygen for generating energy and can rapidly suffer damage. Lacking oxygen, the cells' primary energy supply is lost, as is their ability to generate antioxidants, and they are rapidly subject to oxidation and free radical damage.

Oxygen powers oxidation and reduction (redox) reactions, providing energy and a continuous source of antioxidants. Oxygen is required for generation of energy from the burning of our food in a series of free radical reactions. Absence of oxygen means that these oxidation reactions are interrupted, and sensitive cells, such as those in the brain, rapidly run out of energy. Our bodies run on a series of redox reactions: oxidation removes electrons from molecules and its opposite, reduction by vitamin C and other antioxidants, provides electrons. Tissue damage and death results if this function is prevented, even for a short time.

The heart has four chambers, two collecting chambers (atria) and two pumping chambers (ventricles). The rate of contraction of heart muscle is modified by signals from the nervous system or by hormones such as adrenaline. A specialized section of the nervous system called the autonomic system keeps control of these basic bodily functions without the necessity of conscious attention. Vitamin C protects the autonomic system and is absolutely necessary for the synthesis of adrenaline.[1] Indeed, your body's highest concentrations of ascorbate are found in the adrenal glands.[2] An adequate supply of vitamin C is thus essential for the body to respond appropriately to stress and prevent shock. This action of vitamin C may be one of the main mechanisms for its action in protection against disease, infection, and toxins.[3]

Heart Attacks, Blood Clots, and Strokes

Inappropriate clotting of the blood causes heart attacks and strokes. A blood clot is the result of blood coagulation and is an essential mechanism in the repair of damaged blood vessels. Blood clots are formed when platelets aggregate at the site of an injured blood vessel. While clots are essential to prevent unnecessary blood loss and maintain the integrity of the cardiovascular system, clots occurring at the wrong time or place can block blood vessels, leading to a heart attack. Abnormal blood clotting occurs in conditions that disrupt the normal blood flow. In atrial fibrillation, when the smaller upper chambers of the heart beat rapidly and ineffectively, blood flow slows and clots can form in the stationary blood. Other conditions that can lead to blood clots include heart failure or sitting for long periods on a long flight.

Most people who die of a heart attack seem to enter a period of ventricular fibrillation shortly before death. If a clot in the coronary arteries prevents the blood supply to the heart muscle, the resulting damage can overload the control of ventricular contraction. The wavelike signal to contract is disturbed by the damaged area of the heart wall. As a result, the deflected signal reaches muscle fibers at the wrong time, leading to an uncoordinated contraction. When the ventricles fibrillate, different parts of the main heart muscle contract at dissimilar rates simultaneously and the muscle enters an irregular spasm. These writhing spasms effectively stop the pumping action. Since the cardiac muscle also provides its own blood supply, the muscle can rapidly run out of energy and the ventricles eventually dilate with the resulting relaxation.

Blockage of a vessel supplying the brain will cause an occlusive stroke. Other essential organs with fine capillaries can also be affected, such as a pulmonary embolism blocking the blood supply to a section of lung. These blockages are essentially the same as those occurring in a heart attack or occlusive stroke.

The heart muscle and tissues are supplied by a system of local blood vessels (the left and right coronary arteries). Blood flow through these vessels is largely under local control and responds to increasing demand by raising blood flow. Local hormones, such as the free radical nitric oxide (NO), dilate the coronary arteries. While blocking one of the coronary arteries with a blood clot will rapidly kill or damage the supplied heart muscle, if the blood flow is restricted more slowly, collateral blood vessels may accommodate the change and provide an alternative supply. Small arteries in the heart are often interconnected (anastomosed) and can compensate when minor vessels are blocked. Unfortunately, the larger arteries are independent and blockages are consequently life threatening.

We have a good understanding of the human cardiovascular system as a result of decades of scientific research. A buildup of fat blocking blood flow does not cause heart attacks, as is often erroneously described. Heart attacks and many strokes are a result of a blood clot forming on an inflamed area inside an arterial wall and breaking away to block a coronary vessel. This pathological process depends on a deficiency of vitamin C and related antioxidants.

Atherosclerosis

Atherosclerotic plaques consist of fatty tissues and cells that accumulate within the arterial wall. The early stages of plaque formation involve the attraction of white blood cells and the proliferation of cells in the arterial tissue. Within the developing arterial plaque, cell behavior is disrupted and cholesterol is deposited. Unlike the furring up of water pipes, plaque formation is an active process depending on the response of cells to local injury. Initially, the artery wall responds by thickening locally and expanding in diameter, which keeps the blood flowing as the plaque grows. Thickening of the wall of an artery supplying the heart can prevent it from expanding with increased blood pressure when a person exercises; the result is angina pectoris, a feeling of tightness and pressure in the chest. In other arteries, it can lead to tightening and pain in the legs (intermittent claudication). Eventually, the plaque begins to obstruct the vessel and reduce blood flow; this gradual constriction is called stenosis.

In some cases, the plaque can continue to expand until it totally blocks the artery, preventing the flow of blood. However, only about 15 percent of heart attacks result from direct blockage by a growing plaque; most are caused when the plaque ruptures. Plaques typically cause heart attacks indirectly by causing blood clots.

There are essentially two forms of plaque, stable and unstable. Stable plaques are relatively safe: they may grow slowly and completely block an artery, but this is a rare occurrence. Unstable plaques, as the name implies, are much more dangerous. They have a thin, fibrous cap overlying a soft core of fat and white blood cells, which helps strengthen and contain the plaque's inflamed fat, providing increased stability for a time. But these unstable plaques contain a high level of free radicals, which can lead to splitting of the fibrous cap. Once the cap is damaged, the body attempts to heal this wound as it would attempt to heal any wound—by clotting.

Clotting is a primary mechanism to prevent loss of blood and maintain the integrity of damaged blood vessels.

Plaque-associated clotting can rapidly block the artery. More often, pieces of the clot break free and travel through the bloodstream before coming to rest in an artery too small for the lump to pass through. When this happens in an artery supplying the heart, it deprives the muscle tissue of oxygen and causes a heart attack. Sometimes the clot ends in the brain and kills an area of tissue in an occlusive stroke.

All of the processes leading to a catastrophic event can be slowed or stopped with vitamin C. Heart attacks may simply reflect a shortage in supply of vitamin C and related antioxidants. Dr. William J. McCormick and other early vitamin C researchers first explained the dependency of heart disease on vitamin C levels over half a century ago.[4] This was later elaborated upon by Linus Pauling and others.[5] However, we have yet to see an appropriate research effort into this area despite the alarming levels of atherosclerosis leading to disability and death. Conventional medicine's infatuation with dietary fat and cholesterol has stifled research into vitamin C and heart disease since the middle of the twentieth century.

The Real Cause of Heart Disease— Lifestyle Factors or Inflammation?

Searching for the cause of heart disease involves numerous pathways that end in shortage of vitamin C, inflammation, and oxidative damage. Smoking, high blood pressure, and a high-fat diet may contribute to atherosclerosis, but they are not the cause. Some people will live a long life despite being at high risk from all the major lifestyle risk factors. Others will die early from rampant atherosclerosis but be nonsmoking vegetarians who have a particular aversion to animal fats. The key feature linking the main risk factors is that they produce free radical damage and increase the requirement for vitamin C.

An objection to the idea that conventional risk factors do not explain heart disease might be that genetic factors are also involved. The changing incidence of heart disease in the twentieth century is not explained or reflected by the traditional risk factors, even when considered along with genetic factors.[6] Finding genes for the disease provides pointers to the underlying biochemical problem, but these genes do not by themselves provide an explanation or a therapy. Suggesting the involvement of a genetic component simply means that some people susceptible to heart disease are born with an abnormal biochemistry. However, the human requirement for vitamin C is one of the most ubiquitous genetic abnormalities for our species. The major genetic change in humans—the loss of the ability to synthesize vitamin C—is generally ignored by conventional medicine. But lack of the ability to synthesize vitamin C appears to be the explanation for the human susceptibility to cardiovascular disease.

The concentration on risk factors often obscures the relationship between cardiovascular disease and inflammation. Most risk factors have a pro-inflammatory component. The risk factors for atherosclerosis include disordered lipid (fat) profiles, such as high levels of low-density lipoprotein (LDL) cholesterol in the blood. Autoimmunity and infection are also associated with increased risk, as are high levels of homocysteine, oxidative stress, genetic predisposition, C-reactive protein, and various metabolic diseases.[7] The effects of these risk factors can combine by acting synergistically on separate parts of the inflammatory response. Typically, they stimulate the release of a number of active molecules involved in inflammation, including reactive oxygen species and immune cells that respond to injury.

Risk factors do not directly point to a cause of the disease. They are, however, indicators of inflammation and an increased need for vitamin C. When risk factors are combined, the relative risk increases, which is consistent with the person experiencing chronic inflammation and low-grade scurvy.

The conventional risk factors seem to affect three main cell types that act together in arterial function.[8] Endothelial cells line the inner surface of blood vessels and control flow of hormones and other chemicals into the blood vessel wall.[9] They act as a boundary between the blood vessel and the blood. Deeper in the artery wall, smooth muscle cells maintain the structure and vascular tone of the blood vessel, contracting and expanding to decrease or increase flow. White blood cells can enter the vessel wall to help defend the arteries from chemical and biological insults, but oxidative damage to these white blood cells can result in inflammation of the arterial wall and atherosclerosis. Chronic inflammation in an area of the blood vessel wall interferes with the normal activities of these cells.

Some of the common risk factors for heart disease, such as smoking and high blood pressure, promote oxidation and inflammation in the arterial wall. Oxidation associated with stress can cause white blood cells to adhere to the arterial wall, an early stage of plaque formation.[10] Mechanical and other stresses on the artery produce inflammation and stimulate plaque formation. A sufficient supply of vitamin C is the most important factor in preventing this inflammation and subsequent heart disease. Orthomolecular vitamin C supplementation may be the best way in which an individual can prevent heart disease and stroke. The common factor for the conventional risk factors is their relationship to inflammation and free radical damage. High intakes of vitamin C and related antioxidants can prevent this damage.

It becomes clear that improved prevention and treatment are possible when it is appreciated that atherosclerosis is an inflammatory disease. However, medicine has for decades been transfixed by the idea that cholesterol or other "bad" fats are the underlying cause, even though there was never any hard evidence for this view, merely the presence of cholesterol as a component of the arterial plaque and statistics indicating their association as risk factors. The realization that plaques are areas of an inflamed artery has taken decades to come to the forefront. Inflammation may be considered a rather odd feature to overlook, as inflammation is a characteristic of damaged tissues. Interestingly, persons with inadequate vitamin C are more likely to suffer from both inflammation and high cholesterol.

Plaque inflammation can be active or relatively dormant. Active plaques with acute inflammation are the most dangerous. Plaques can remain dormant for years but flare up occasionally to put the person at risk of clot formation, heart attack, or stroke. Often, inflammation in plaques is associated with infection. Many drugs currently in use for the treatment of heart disease, such as aspirin and the statins, have anti-inflammatory, antioxidant, or antimicrobial properties, although they are often given for other reasons.[11] Most of the conventional risk factors for heart disease and stroke cause inflammation and free radical damage. The transition of the low-grade inflammation of a dormant plaque to the active dangerous form occurs when there are insufficient antioxidants. High intakes of vitamin C may prevent this transition and prevent heart attacks completely.

The body constantly requires vitamin C to repair minor damage to its tissues. In the case of atherosclerosis, the repair mechanisms fail. This failure is a direct result of a lack of available antioxidants, particularly vitamin C. Risk factors for heart disease and stroke relate in some way to the arterial disease or its progress, but they are not the cause of the illness. The focus on supposed risk factors, such as cholesterol, reflects an ignorance of the underlying biological processes. This focus ignores the finding that animals that synthesize vitamin C internally are resistant to atherosclerosis.[12] Humans may achieve a corresponding freedom from cardiovascular disease by supplementing with high, dynamic flow levels of vitamin C.

The Process of Atherosclerosis

Any chemical, mechanical, or immunological insult to an artery produces free radical damage. This damage triggers a cascade of inflammatory reactions aimed at local repair, the activation of the immune system, and a massive local increased need for antioxidants. The result is a local area of

Blood Pressure: Risk or Explanation?

Risk factors such as cholesterol do not explain the location of plaques within the arterial system. Mechanical and other stresses on the artery produce inflammation and stimulate plaque formation. Plaques occur more frequently in places that are stressed—often near the heart, where blood vessels stretch and bend. High blood pressure and pulsating blood flow tend to flex the vessels in these areas. The flow of blood around an obstruction also causes mechanical stress as the blood shears along the inner lining of the artery. In the case of high blood pressure, there is a simple mechanical relationship between the "risk factor" and damage to the arterial wall. This mechanism explains at least part of the distribution of arterial damage and plaques in cardiovascular disease.

Blood pressure is controlled by several mechanisms, including nerves and hormones, but the detailed controls are not completely understood. Systolic pressure is the peak pressure in the arteries and corresponds to the contraction of the heart muscle. The diastolic pressure is the lowest pressure and corresponds to the relaxation of the heart muscle. Normal ranges of blood pressure in the adult are typically assumed to be:

• Systolic: 90–135 mm Hg   • Diastolic: 70–90 mm Hg

Children tend to have lower pressures, while in the elderly the measurements are typically higher. The increase in the elderly may result from reduced flexibility of the arteries, but this is not necessarily a consequence of normal aging. Not everyone experiences inflammation in which almost all of the traditional risk factors may play a minor part.

Atherosclerosis appears to start with a minor disruption or damage to the blood vessel wall when vitamin C is in short supply. The damage begins with endothelial cells that separate the blood from the arterial wall.[14] These cells sense the current conditions and provide signals to control the healing response of the artery, maintain blood vessel tone, and maintain blood flow.[15] Endothelial cells control the flow of nutrients to the artery wall and are intimately involved in the initiation of inflammation.

When injured, the endothelial cells release a number of molecules (fibronectin, selectins, interleukin-1, intracellular adhesion molecule, vascular cell adhesion molecule, and others) that signal monocyte white blood cells in the blood to penetrate the blood vessel wall. Specific signals to initiate

increasing blood pressure with age, so the condition may be an indication of chronic shortage of vitamin C, magnesium, and other nutrients in the modern diet.

Typical values for a healthy young adult at rest are usually given as 120 mm Hg systolic and 80 mm Hg diastolic ("120 over 80"), but there are large individual variations. Values above 120/80 are potentially pre-hypertensive and dietary modification may be considered. Some people have higher values, some lower, and some have a variation in the difference between the measured pressures. Furthermore, the measured values vary rapidly throughout the day with time and conditions in a single individual. They also change in response to numerous factors, such as stress, nutrition, and disease. This stress response can lead to the "white coat" effect—higher values being found by doctors and other staff in clinical settings. Such increased pressures can lead to people being unnecessarily worried, or overmedicated, for a condition they do not have. A person concerned about possible hypertension should monitor their pressure with readings taken at the same time over a period of days or weeks. Blood pressure measurement is often unreliable.

When uncontrolled, high blood pressure can result in aneurysms, in which an artery balloons out like a weak spot on an inner tube. Alternatively, repeated stress can cause chronic local inflammation, generating an arterial plaque of scarlike tissue in an attempt to repair the damage.[13] High blood pressure is often described as a "risk factor" for heart disease, but for once there is a clear causal relationship between the "risk factor" of blood pressure and localized arterial stress.

an inflammatory response may also be released.[16] Factors that affect blood clotting (thromboxane, von Willebrand factor, prostacyclin, and tissue plasminogen) may also be produced.[17] One of the more important local hormones regulating vascular tone and blood flow is nitric oxide (NO), which is released by the endothelial cells. NO is a free radical used extensively by our cells as a chemical signal in the control of local blood flow and blood pressure.[18] It typically acts to dilate and increase flow and is thus antagonistic to other better-known hormones, such as adrenaline.[19] In order to function properly and maintain healthy vessels and blood flow, nitric oxide is dependent on adequate amounts of vitamin C.[20]

With an adequate supply of vitamin C, the epithelial cells can increase production of NO when the blood vessel wall is stressed or damaged.[21] NO production is signaled by several chemical factors (acetylcholine, thromboxane, bradykinin, estrogen, substance P, histamine, insulin, bacterial endotoxins, and adenosine) and mechanical factors, such as the shear stress of the blood flow.[22] Nitric oxide is a gas that can dissolve in and diffuse readily through water and fat. This molecule will dilate blood vessels. NO is an essential early part of the defense mechanism of the arterial wall. People who have a defective nitric oxide response, resulting from vitamin C deficiency, can suffer increased resistance to blood flow and thickening of the blood vessel wall.

In 2003, American pharmacologist Louis J. Ignarro, Ph.D., suggested that atherosclerotic plaques act like trash caught in a river bend, impeding the flow. The result is local stress on the epithelial wall of the artery. Dr. Ignarro proposed that treatment with vitamin C and other antioxidants (vitamin E and alpha-lipoic acid) together with the amino acid L-arginine could prevent blood vessel inflammation and subsequent damage. He received the 1998 Nobel Prize in Physiology or Medicine for his work on nitric oxide signaling in the cardiovascular system. His experiments suggested that dietary supplements of antioxidant vitamins and L-arginine could lower the risk of heart disease in mice.[23] He believed this vitamin C–based approach would produce similar results in patients with heart disease.[24]

When smooth muscle cells within arteries contract, they reduce the diameter of the vessel and help maintain vascular tone and blood pressure. Unlike skeletal muscle, smooth muscle cells are not normally under conscious control. The autonomic nervous system and hormones such as adrenaline provide smooth muscle tone as well as the elasticity necessary for dissipating the energy of blood flow pulses arising from the beating of the heart. In people with high blood pressure or with atherosclerosis, the smooth muscle cells can secrete local hormones and other active chemicals, which attract white blood cells and act as growth promoters.[25] This change is thought to add to the strength of the developing arterial plaque.[26] As the smooth muscle cells proliferate, they secrete proteins that combine with collagen and elastic fibers to form a fibrous cap over the advancing plaque.[27]

As the plaque grows and develops, there is an increased cholesterol and lipid content. The smooth muscle cells in advanced plaques appear aged and have increased rates of cell death. These cells are more sensitive to damage by free radicals and may be killed by white blood cells activated by the local inflammation. The death of these muscle cells can further stimulate the inflammatory process, weakening the arterial wall and causing it to balloon out as an aneurysm.[28] If the fibrous cap ruptures, it releases fats and fragments of plaque into the bloodstream and is recognized by the blood as a wound (lesion). The blood responds by forming a clot to seal off the damaged blood vessel wall.[29] With small plaque ruptures, the tissue may partially heal, including clot material into the plaque. Larger plaque ruptures can lead to clots that block the artery. Prevention of plaque rupture with orthomolecular levels of vitamin C could provide an effective prevention of heart attack and stroke.

White blood cells are a component of inflammation and their contribution to atherosclerosis is expected. Monocyte white blood cells migrate from the blood into the arterial wall, ultimately leading to further oxidative damage to the epithelial cells. When activated by injury, the endothelial cells cause monocytes to stick to the interior surface of the artery. The monocytes then squeeze through the gaps between the endothelial cells and enter the arterial wall. As the plaque develops further, more monocytes are recruited with the release of local hormones from cells in the inflamed tissue. Once in the plaque, monocytes can transform into another type of white blood cell called macrophages, which engulf microscopic foreign bodies as part of the immune response. Reactive oxygen species, typically present in inflammation, signal the change from monocyte to macrophage.[30]

In the absence of sufficient vitamin C, the inflammation continues and the activity of the macrophages may cease to be beneficial and cause the plaque to rupture. Once inside the plaque, macrophages help the repair process by taking up lipoproteins, such as LDL cholesterol, including those that have been oxidized or otherwise degraded. The oxidized cholesterol is, however, toxic and can damage the macrophage.[31] Macrophages take lipids within their bodies, but if this accumulation becomes extreme, the interiors of the cells starts to look foamy and they are called "foam cells." Foam cells often die within the plaque from apoptosis. They are considered harmful and a potential source of additional oxygen radicals.[32] Macrophages accumulate in the core of the plaque as it ages, and this accumulation is associated with a softening of the plaque, increasing risk of plaque rupture and heart attack.[33] Each stage of this pathological process depends on oxidation and free radical damage, suggesting a local deficit in antioxidants.

Is Heart Disease Infectious?

The role of infectious agents in common diseases in humans, such as heart disease and stomach ulcers, has been downplayed by conventional medicine. However, since the discovery that peptic ulcers are caused by *Helicobacter pylori*, we might expect the idea that other common long-term diseases are caused by infections to be given serious consideration.[34] Vitamin C is a powerful antiviral, antibacterial, and immune-stimulating agent. It would therefore be predicted to prevent or eliminate heart disease under this model. The idea that heart disease might be an infection was suggested early in the twentieth century and is now being reconsidered because traditional risk factors do not explain the cause of the disease.[35]

There are a number of potential candidates for infectious agents that cause heart disease, including influenza A and B, adenovirus, enterovirus, coxsackie B4 virus, and various herpes viruses (especially cytomegalovirus). Viruses are known to infect the cells of blood vessels[36] and atherosclerotic areas may be more available for viral attack.[37] Bacterial infections with *Chlamydia pneumoniae, H. pylori, Hemophilus influenzae, Mycoplasma pneumoniae, Mycobacterium tuberculosis,* and gingivitis may also be involved.[38] Multiple disease organisms can be found, such as those also found in gum disease (*Porphyromonas gingivalis* and *Streptococcus sanguis*), and the infection could provide a trigger for acute events resulting in clot formation.[39] Multiple organisms can act together to give increased inflammation or a modified plaque.[40] The available evidence suggests that the overall microbial burden is linked to opportunistic infection of the arteries and heart attack.[41]

Infection acts to speed up the process of inflammatory damage, as opportunistic viral and other organisms can give rise to increased oxidation and free radical damage.[42] The idea that atherosclerosis is an infection is a scientifically reasonable hypothesis, and we can be fairly certain that if an infection produces or contributes to chronic local inflammation in an artery, a plaque will result. Both viral and bacterial infections aggravate lesion development in animal models of atherosclerosis.[43] More importantly, perhaps, is the variability in host susceptibility to the pathogens, which appears to relate to the ability to generate a successful immune response and, particularly, control inflammation.

Herpes

In the 1970s, researchers found that a bird virus, called Marek's disease herpes virus (MDV), caused atherosclerosis in chickens. The involvement of viruses in the progression of the disease in birds may be indirect by stimulation of the immune system generating a local inflammatory response.[44] The resulting plaques had fibrous, thickening, and atherosclerotic changes similar to those found in human disease.[45] Striking plaques were seen in large coronary arteries, aortas, and major aortic branches of chickens with both normal and high cholesterol levels. Uninfected chickens had no large plaques, whether or not they were fed high-cholesterol diets. Notably the development of atherosclerosis in these chickens could be prevented by immunization against herpes virus.[46]

By the 1980s, scientists were beginning to take the idea of atherosclerosis as an infectious disease seriously. The atherosclerotic plaques in Japanese quail were examined and herpes DNA was consistently found in the aortas of embryos selected for genetic susceptibility to atherosclerosis but in a far smaller fraction of unsusceptible quail embryos.[47] These results suggest that genetic susceptibility to atherosclerosis in birds may be linked to an immune deficiency or viral genes being passed through the generations. Later research demonstrated that rats infected with herpes also developed blood vessel lesions[48] and mice infected with herpes are more susceptible to atherosclerosis.[49]

When atherosclerotic plaques in humans were examined for herpes simplex DNA, it was present.[50] DNA from other herpes viruses, such as cytomegalovirus, are also found within arteries in humans and is associated with atherosclerotic plaques.[51] This virus also may be linked to aortic aneurysms in humans.[52] Until 1995, active virus had not been isolated from atherosclerotic plaque, but a decade later it had been found associated with specific cell types.[53] However, a latent virus can lie dormant for years until the immune system is unable to keep it in check. Latent herpes virus, waiting to infect people with weakened immune systems, is known to be common, especially in patients with atherosclerosis.[54] Both the smooth muscle cells in arteries and white blood cells attracted to sites of arterial damage are candidates for harboring the virus.[55] Immunosuppressed patients with herpes infection are prone to atherosclerosis; an infection with cytomegalovirus is also associated with reduced long-term survival in heart transplant patients.[56] That heart transplants in children often fail through atherosclerotic changes appears quite inconsistent with the idea of lifestyle risk factors being the primary cause.[57]

Periodically activated virus may have a role in the pathogenesis of atherosclerosis. When the arteries of young trauma victims were examined, herpes virus was found both in normal sections of artery and in early atherosclerotic lesions.[58] Since herpes viruses have been implicated in the initiation and development of atherosclerosis, it could be that immunization against these would prevent the disease.[59] However, cytomegalovirus damages coronary arteries by a progressive inflammatory response that involves proliferation of smooth muscle cells. Inhibition of this cell proliferation can be obtained using antioxidants, suggesting that oxidative stress following viral exposure might be triggering the proliferation.[60] If several infective agents are involved, vaccination against a specific organism would be futile. The available evidence suggests that high doses of vitamin C will prevent a wide range of infective agents and thus be more effective.

Chlamydia

Most people know *Chlamydia trachomatis* as the cause of a common sexually transmitted disease. Most people with chlamydia have no symptoms and are unaware of the infection; it is also a frequent cause of preventable blindness in many parts of the world. However, with heart disease, we are mainly concerned with another form of chlamydia, *Chlamydia pneumoniae*. *Chlamydia pneumoniae* is a microorganism that infects the respiratory tract and is also claimed to be involved in atherosclerosis.[61]

It is transmitted person-to-person in the air with respiratory secretions. All ages are at risk of infection but it is most common in school-age children. About half of all adults in the United States have evidence of infection by age twenty. It has been estimated that it causes about 10 percent of all community-acquired pneumonia in adults and 5 percent of bronchitis and sinusitis. However, most infections with this organism do not produce symptoms but infections can flare up, causing common and important respiratory tract diseases. Re-infection remains common throughout life.

The association of heart disease with Chlamydia appears solidly based on the available evidence.[62] In young adults, this organism is found in association with arterial plaques more frequently than in normal arterial wall, and there is some evidence that antibodies may be present in the blood early in atherosclerosis.[63] Furthermore, Chlamydia has been found in arterial disease when no antibodies were apparent in the blood.[64] Other researchers have found antibodies against both Chlamydia and cytomegalovirus to be linked with early and advanced carotid atherosclerosis.[65]

But the evidence linking Chlamydia and atherosclerosis is not fully consistent.[66] If atherosclerosis is a result of infection caused by chronic shortage of vitamin C, this lack of consistency is expected: the infection involved in a particular case may simply reflect which virus, or bacteria, was available to infect the tissue. Chlamydia DNA is found in a high proportion of cardiac transplant patients, and higher numbers of antibodies in the blood may be linked with the abnormally rapid atherosclerosis and failure of the transplant.[67] The accumulation of evidence linking Chlamydia with atherosclerosis is convincing[68] but does not necessarily indicate that it is a dominant cause of the disease.[69]

Chlamydia has been demonstrated to cause atherosclerosis in animal experiments, which can be prevented by antibiotic treatment.[70] A preliminary study with antibiotics on atherosclerotic patients with Chlamydia suggested a decrease in acute coronary events in a month.[71] Unlike vitamin C, however, antibiotics are not effective against viruses, do not modulate the inflammatory process, and do not directly aid healing. Chlamydia can act as a local oxidant and free radical generator. It can oxidize cholesterol-related molecules, a process considered to be an essential part of plaque development.[72] High-dose vitamin C can prevent such oxidation, protecting the arterial wall.

While the association of Chlamydia with atherosclerosis is established, it is not clear whether it is causative or an opportunistic infection. Its involvement may depend on a shortage of vitamin C and pre-existing damage to the artery. Chlamydia may just be the most commonly available infection for invading damaged arteries. An alternative approach to antibiotics would be to boost the immune response with adequate amounts of vitamin C and prevent the infection occurring.

Other Infective Agents

Antibodies to both herpes and Epstein-Barr virus are often increased in patients with atherosclerosis. The viruses are found separately and in combined infection. Epstein-Barr virus was recently shown to be present in atherosclerotic plaques along with *Herpes simplex* and cytomegalovirus.[73] However, some subjects with atherosclerosis show no antibodies to either virus.[74]

The human immunodeficiency virus (HIV) implicated in AIDS is associated with suppression of the immune response. Patients infected with HIV have an increased rate of development of atherosclerosis.[75] The resulting arterial lesions are intermediate in structure between normal plaque and transplant disease. Some findings indicate the possible involvement of *Mycobacterium tuberculosis,* the organism that causes TB, in atherosclerosis.[76] High levels of *Mycobacteria*-related protein can be found in animal studies and in atherosclerotic patients. Moreover, atherosclerotic changes can be found in the vascular wall of animals vaccinated with *Mycobacteria*-related protein.

The presence of organisms in plaques that are usually found in gingivitis is informative. Infected gums potentially present a range of microorganisms to the bloodstream and thus to the arteries. Damaged arteries might be easy and inviting targets to such infection. Several bacteria (*Bacteroides forsythus, Porphyromonas gingivalis, Actinobacillus actinomycetemcomitans,* and *Prevotella intermedia*) found in diseased gums have also been found in arterial plaque.[77] However, studies on the association between cardiovascular disease and periodontal disease or loss of teeth have produced conflicting results.[78] The presence of gingivitis may indicate an increased risk of atherosclerosis, but the effect may be relatively small.[79]

Vitamin C and the Antioxidant Defense of Heart Disease

Human plaque might contain more vitamins C and E than is found in healthy arteries. In plaques, however, both vitamin E and coenzyme Q_{10} are oxidized.[80] These antioxidants require a constant re-supply of electrons in order to prevent free radical damage.[81] As Dr. Robert F. Cathcart III points out, effective antioxidant treatment of disease needs a massive intake of vitamin C to supply antioxidant electrons. Under the inflammatory conditions within a plaque, normal metabolism is insufficient to provide these reducing electrons. Few dietary antioxidants can provide a free supply of antioxidant electrons to such tissue—the exception is vitamin C under conditions of dynamic flow. Plaques that are in an oxidized state could, in principle, be rendered healthy with sufficient vitamin C.[82]

The Importance of Nitric Oxide

As we have explained, nitric oxide works with vitamin C in maintaining healthy blood vessels. Damage to the synthesis of this small molecule may be one of the first steps leading to atherosclerosis.[83] It is formed from the amino acid arginine and the enzyme nitric oxide synthetase catalyzes the reaction. The manufacture of nitric oxide also involves vitamins B_2 (riboflavin) and B_3 (niacin).[84] Once formed, nitric oxide diffuses through the endothelial cell membrane into the smooth muscle of the arterial wall. Inside the artery, it helps control vascular tone.

Under oxidizing conditions, superoxide can be produced instead of nitric oxide.[85] Superoxide is also generated during inflammation (white blood cells activated by inflammation release superoxide) and will quench nitric oxide and prevent it from relaxing and dilating the local arterial wall. As inflammation develops, superoxide will directly constrict local blood vessels, further antagonizing the action of NO. Vitamin C at high concentration can prevent such oxidative damage to the arteries and restore the beneficial role of nitric oxide.[86]

Nitric oxide is a central part of many normal and disease processes, including inflammation, infection, and regulation of blood pressure. The roles of NO, like other redox active species, depend on the local tissue and its environment. Too much nitric oxide can contribute to vascular cell pathology, killing cells and producing free radical damage.[87] Exceptionally high levels of NO can damage brain cells when the blood supply is inadequate. Conversely, release of nitric oxide from endothelial cells can reduce injury from lack of blood flow by dilating the blood vessel. Low NO in tissues, or decreased sensitivity to its effects, impairs the ability of arteries to expand when required and increases the ability of atherosclerosis to produce clinical illness.[88] In advanced atherosclerosis, arteries may produce less nitric oxide, which may be related to the presence of oxidized cholesterol and other free radicals.[89]

A high level of antioxidants, and particularly vitamin C, are necessary for nitric oxide to protect the blood vessels, especially in people with conventional risk factors for atherosclerosis. Nitric oxide may inhibit the proliferation of smooth muscle cells in the blood vessel wall, which occurs in atherosclerosis. When tissue levels of oxidants are high, as in an inflamed arterial wall, NO production may be high but ineffective. Shock, generalized inflammation, and bacterial toxins can increase the synthesis of NO and induce hypotension. Clinical reports beginning sixty years ago with Dr. Frederick R. Klenner suggest that sufficiently high levels of vitamin C can prevent this pathology. Several antioxidants appear to be able to quench free radicals and preserve nitric oxide's function in blood vessels. These antioxidants include vitamins C and E,[90] alpha-lipoic acid,[91] coenzyme Q_{10},[92] glutathione,[93] superoxide dismutase (SOD),[94] selenium,[95] and quercetin.[96] However, the antioxidant function of vitamin C is unique in providing a driving potential promoting the actions of these other antioxidants.[97]

Antioxidant Network Therapy

The well-known five-a-day portions of fruits and vegetables is aimed at increasing the intake of antioxidants and phytochemicals. This recommendation may have originated as the requirement to achieve conventional, Recommended Dietary Allowance (RDA) levels of vitamin C. However, the recommendation is at best misleading, and at worst it promises more than it can deliver. The biggest problem with "five-a-day" is that this intake is clearly inadequate to provide sufficient antioxidants to compensate for the modern diet of fast food and abnormal fats. There has been a dramatic loss of nutrients in vegetables over the last half century, caused by changes in variety, storage, and preservation. This may also be due to intensive farming and chemical fertilizers (organic foods typically contain more nutrients). The government recommendations do not appear to take full account of the decline in nutrients in our food, reducing the availability of food with high levels of vitamin C and other nutrients.

High-dose vitamin C and other antioxidants is the only answer. High-dose vitamin C can inhibit atherosclerosis in animals even in the presence of high blood cholesterol. There is supporting evidence on the benefits of antioxidants in humans from epidemiology and clinical trials.[98] Low levels of quercetin, for example, may be associated with increased death from heart attack.[99] Alpha-lipoic acid has a strong anti-inflammatory action on damaged arterial walls[100] and induces production of nitric oxide. However, studies on humans have generally used low doses and inappropriate antioxidant supplements and give conflicting results.[101]

Vitamin C drives the capability of numerous other antioxidants, such as alpha-lipoic acid, vitamin E, and coenzyme Q_{10}. This simple vitamin is at the core of an antioxidant network that protects the body from damage and ill health. Following from the early work of Linus Pauling and others, orthomolecular nutrition has derived an antioxidant network therapy based on the central role of vitamin C.

Prevention of heart disease appears to require a minimum of about 3 grams of vitamin C, in doses spread throughout the day. In general, this should be taken along with a high-quality orthomolecular multivitamin. A broad range of additional dietary antioxidants, such as vitamin E and selenium, would also be beneficial. People at higher risk can increase their intake of vitamin C and add specific antioxidants. The most useful additional antioxidants appear to be vitamin E (mixed natural tocotrienols combined with extra tocopherols) and alpha-lipoic acid. All these antioxidants are widely available from health food stores. Dr. Pauling and others have also proposed the addition of amino acids, such as lysine, proline, arginine, and citrulline. These substances have low toxicity, may be beneficial, and help vitamin C prevent arterial inflammation.

Antioxidant network therapy to prevent heart disease might include the following supplements daily:

- Vitamin C, at or near bowel tolerance (6+ grams)
- Lysine, 3–6 grams
- Proline, 0.5–2.0 grams
- Arginine, 3.5 grams
- Citrulline, 1.5 grams
- Mixed tocotrienols (vitamin E), 300+ mg
- Mixed tocopherols (vitamin E), 800+ IU
- R-alpha-lipoic acid, 300–600 mg

To remove existing atherosclerotic plaques and return a person with pre-existing heart disease to good health is more difficult than preventing the illness. These suggested doses of vitamin C are probably too small for clinical benefit in that case—the bowel tolerance method of dosing, proposed by Dr. Cathcart, is more appropriate (*see* Chapter 3). The resulting vitamin C dose will vary with the individual, between, say, 10 and 30 grams per day. In cases of existing disease, a minimum of six months of treatment with antioxidant network therapy is needed before any reduction in plaque size would be expected. A maximal effect might take two to three years. However, even subjects with advanced atherosclerosis can stabilize and reduce plaques, preventing heart attack and stroke.

Vitamin C is the key factor, whether heart disease is caused by inflammation, infection, oxidation, fats, or poor lifestyle. This single vitamin protects against the core aspects of the pathology. There are many factors that can initiate minor local damage in the arterial wall, such as poor nutrition and high blood pressure. Chronic infection appears to promote the development of atherosclerosis: while it might not produce the initial lesion, infection can accelerate the development of plaque by promoting local inflammation. Any area of damage in the body and the resulting inflammation is an opportunity for colonization by a microorganism. The role of the microorganism may be to infect, grow, and rupture plaques more quickly than would otherwise be the case.

People with well-functioning immune systems based on an optimal intake of vitamin C may have a distinct advantage and avoid the ravages of heart disease. Heart disease may eventually be shown to be an infectious disease, where the infection takes hold when there is insufficient vitamin C to repair arterial damage. Vitamin C supplementation may be the simplest way of boosting the immune system to prevent atherosclerosis and stroke. High levels of vitamin C are needed to prevent vascular damage and facilitate repair of the tissues. Dynamic flow levels of vitamin C are claimed to prevent infection taking hold. As evidence accumulates, it is clear that shortage of vitamin C appears increasingly likely to be the ultimate cause of heart disease.

The good news is that abundant ascorbate may also provide a cure.

Conclusion

*"Actually, we can make more ascorbate than a dog, cat, or rat,
but in our chemical plants; we just have to have the brains to
know how to take the massive doses necessary in acute situations."*
—ROBERT F. CATHCART III, M.D.

The vitamin C story stretches back to the early evolution of our human ancestors. Because of a prehistoric genetic error, scurvy has plagued humans throughout history, whenever dietary vitamin C was in short supply. It is only in the last hundred years that scientists have isolated vitamin C and identified it as ascorbic acid, a simple organic molecule. A few milligrams of this inexpensive white powder will prevent or cure acute scurvy. Scurvy still occurs, though doctors sometimes misdiagnose it as a severe infection, because the acute disease has become rare and unusual.

Human evolution has been marked by periods of environmental crises, in which the population appears to have crashed. At times, only a few thousand early humans may have remained. These people were probably under dietary stress, through food shortage and starvation. Surprisingly, people and animals that do not manufacture ascorbate within their systems might have a survival advantage when food is short. Since they did not use essential glucose and energy to synthesize vitamin C, these people may have saved the energy equivalent of a small cup of milk each day. Thus, if we had not lost the gene for vitamin C, our species may not have survived.

In recent times, with the gradual extension of life expectancy, people have experienced an increased incidence of chronic disease. However, thousands of years ago, as our ancestors struggled to survive and repro-

143

duce, such diseases were irrelevant compared to finding food and not being eaten by predators. Few prehistoric people lived long enough to suffer the chronic diseases of old age.

For decades, nutritionally aware doctors have suggested that chronic diseases, such as heart disease, arthritis, and cancer, are now common because we have too low an intake of vitamin C. These physicians have made astounding claims for the effectiveness of vitamin C against these diseases. However, conventional medicine has ignored such clinical reports, or explained them away as wishful thinking or the placebo effect. Despite this, reports continue, though they are not followed up with the clinical trials we might expect. A cynical view is that there are scant profits to be made from nutrition compared with those from drugs and related treatments.

Conventional and Orthomolecular Nutrition

The science of nutrition falls into two categories, conventional and orthomolecular. Conventional nutritionists (also known as dieticians, particularly in health settings) consider that vitamins are micronutrients, required in small quantities. Orthomolecular practitioners suggest that higher doses are needed for optimal health. According to the conventional view, supplemental vitamins or nutrients offer few health benefits and may, supposedly, even cause harm. The general message seems to be that, provided we consume a balanced diet, cut down on fats, and eat fruits and vegetables, we will all enjoy optimal health.

Orthomolecular nutritionists consider that nutrition is the primary factor in good health rather than being merely peripheral to drug-based or surgical interventions. They realize that the available information on vitamin C and other nutrients is incomplete. Nevertheless, using vitamin C in high doses, they report that it has a powerful antiviral action, prevents heart disease, and, in large enough doses, is selectively toxic to cancer cells. Orthomolecular medicine is full of promise and excitement and provides a way to break through the major problems facing conventional medicine, and each of us.

Not the End but the Future

We have followed the story of vitamin C from its evolutionary beginnings to its identification as ascorbic acid in the early years of the twentieth century. Its classification as a vitamin confused conventional medicine into a rigid paradigm, in which only milligram amounts were deemed "necessary." However, since its isolation, some doctors and scientists have been arguing that people need larger amounts. These doctors were ignored and censored, despite reporting effects for very large doses of vitamin C that are unparalleled in medicine.

The great chemist Linus Pauling put his massive scientific reputation behind the vitamin, after claiming that it might help prevent or treat the common cold. Dr. Pauling's cold-cure claim caused him to be branded a quack and charlatan. Since then, the public has been made aware of the strange claims and story behind vitamin C, even though the media and medical establishment have done virtually nothing to tell the real story of ascorbate. One way they have deceived the public is by telling them that a gram (1,000 mg) of vitamin C each day is a "high dose" and then reporting that such a "high" dose has no effect on colds or other illnesses. We agree that a gram of vitamin C each day will have little beneficial effect on a cold, but would add that it would be supportive of good health. However, the idea that a gram is a high dose is simply absurd.

Indeed, vitamin C studies have usually involved doses 50–100 times too small, taken at intervals perhaps ten times too long. We have been told that the effects of vitamin C are small and thus only studies that include a placebo control can be considered valid. This is wrong. The claims for high-dose vitamin C are among the strongest scientific hypotheses possible in clinical medicine. The humble placebo could not cause such large effects.

In recounting the story of vitamin C, we have taken a meandering route, including accounts of several physicians and scientists whose work is central to the plot. We have also covered the way science has evolved from an experimental and clinical discipline to what today is almost a branch of sociology dominated by statistical analysis. Without an appreciation of how modern medicine has generated the myth that the placebo has superpowers, it would be difficult to see how this has been used to suppress the direct clinical reports of the effects of vitamin C.

We cannot predict what vitamin C's status will be ten years from now. Public interest in vitamin C is strong and growing—vitamin C is the most commonly taken vitamin supplement. Yet, the powerful lobbying of the pharmaceutical giants, together with the conservatism of physicians and scientists, may mean that it will remain largely untested in sufficiently high doses. Currently, it looks as if the benefits of intravenous sodium ascorbate in cancer might start to be exploited. However, this will likely involve vitamin C given alone or alongside conventional chemotherapy. In this way, the larger potential benefits of redox synergy between vitamin C and other nutrients, such as alpha-lipoic acid or forms of selenium, will remain hidden from view.

One day soon the practice of medicine may be revolutionized by an appreciation of the beneficial effects of high-dose vitamin C. The only thing preventing such progress is the refusal of medical science to perform the necessary clinical trials. Vitamin C is only one of many nutrients that can potentially provide incredible health benefits when taken in orthomolecular doses.

Soon perhaps, health care without high-dose nutrient therapy will be considered to be like childbirth without sanitation or surgery without anesthetic. But can we afford to wait?

References

INTERNET RESOURCES

Journal of Orthomolecular Medicine (free full-text papers)
http://orthomolecular.org/library/jom/

Oregon State University's Linus Pauling Institute
http://lpi.oregonstate.edu/

Frederick R. Klenner's book *Clinical Guide to the Use of Vitamin C*
www.seanet.com/~alexs/ascorbate/198x/smith-lh-clinical_guide_1988.htm

C for Yourself
www.cforyourself.com

Vitamin C Foundation
www.vitamincfoundation.org/

Ascorbate Web
www.seanet.com/~alexs/ascorbate

Irwin Stone's book *The Healing Factor: Vitamin C Against Disease*
http://vitamincfoundation.org/stone/

REFERENCES

Chapter 1: A Remarkable Molecule

1. Carr, A.C., and B. Frei. "Toward a New Recommended Dietary Allowance for Vitamin C Based on Antioxidant and Health Effects in Humans." *Am J Clin Nutr* 69:6 (1999): 1086–1107.

2. Simon, J.A., and E.S. Hudes. "Serum Ascorbic Acid and Gallbladder Disease Prevalence among U.S. Adults: The Third National Health and Nutrition Examination Survey (NHANES III)." *Arch Intern Med* 160:7 (2000): 931–936.

3. Meister, A. "Glutathione-ascorbic Acid Antioxidant System in Animals." *J Biol Chem* 269:13 (1994): 9397–9400.

4. Meister, A. "On the Antioxidant Effects of Ascorbic Acid and Glutathione." *Biochem Pharmacol* 44 (1992): 1905–1915.

5. Mårtensson, J.M., J. Han, O.W. Griffith, et al. "Glutathione Ester Delays the Onset of Scurvy in Ascorbate-deficient Guinea Pigs." *Proc Natl Acad Sci USA* 90 (1993): 317–321.

6. Montecinos, V., P. Guzmán, V. Barra, et al. "Vitamin C is an Essential Antioxidant that Enhances Survival of Oxidatively Stressed Human Vascular Endothelial Cells in the Presence of a Vast Molar Excess of Glutathione." *J Biol Chem* 282:21 (2007): 15506–15515.

7. Cancer Research U.K. "U.K. Failing to Eat 5 a Day." Press release, September 21, 2007.

8. Gadsby, P. "The Inuit Paradox: How Can People Who Gorge on Fat and Rarely See a Vegetable Be Healthier than We Are?" *Discover Magazine* (January 10, 2004). Bell, R.A., E.J. Mayer-Davis, Y. Jackson, et al. "An Epidemiologic Review of Dietary Intake Studies among American Indians and Alaska Natives: Implications for Heart Disease and Cancer Risk." *Ann Epidemiol* 7:4 (1997): 229–240.

9. Hansen, J.C., H.S. Pedersen, G. Mulvad. "Fatty Acids and Antioxidants in the Inuit Diet. Their Role in Ischemic Heart Disease (IHD) and Possible Interactions with Other Dietary Factors. A Review." *Arctic Med Res* 53:1 (1994): 4–17.

10. Lewis, H.W. *Why Flip a Coin?* New York, NY: John Wiley and Sons, 1997.

11. Stone, I. "The Natural History of Ascorbic Acid in the Evolution of the Mammals and Primates and Its Significance for Present Day Man." *Orthomolecular Psych* 1:2–3 (1972): 82–89. Stone, I. "Fifty Years of Research on Ascorbate and the Genetics of Scurvy." *J Orthomolecular Psych* 13:3 (1984).

Available online at: www.orthomed.org/resources/papers/stnwnd.htm. Stone, I. "Studies of a Mammalian Enzyme System for Producing Evolutionary Evidence on Man." *Am J Phys Anthropol* 23 (1965): 83–86.

12. Pauling, L. "Evolution and the Need for Ascorbic Acid." *Proc Natl Acad Sci USA* 67 (1970): 1643–1648.

13. Pigolotti, S., A. Flammini, M. Marsili, et al. "Species Lifetime Distribution for Simple Models of Ecologies." *Proc Natl Acad Sci USA* 102:44 (2005): 15747–15751. Newman, M.E.J., and R.G. Palmer. *Modeling Extinction.* New York, NY: Oxford University Press, 2003.

14. Reich, D.E., and D.B. Goldstein. "Genetic Evidence for a Paleolithic Human Population Expansion in Africa." *Proc Natl Acad Sci USA* 95:14 (1998): 8119–8123.

15. Sykes, B. *Seven Daughters of Eve: The Science That Reveals Our Genetic Ancestry.* New York, NY: W.W. Norton, 2001. Fay, J.C, and C.I. Wu. "A Human Population Bottleneck Can Account for the Discordance between Patterns of Mitochondrial versus Nuclear DNA Variation." *Mol Biol Evol* 16:7 (1999): 1003–1005.

16. Cann, R.L., M. Stoneking, A.C. Wilson. "Mitochondrial DNA and Human Evolution." *Nature* 325 (1987): 31–36.

17. Ambrose, S. "Did the Super-eruption of Toba Cause a Human Population Bottleneck? Reply to Gathorne-Hardy and Harcourt-Smith." *J Hum Evol* 45 (2003): 231–237. Ambrose, S. "Late Pleistocene Human Population Bottlenecks, Volcanic Winter, and the Differentiation of Modern Humans." *J Hum Evol* 34 (1998): 623–651.

18. Feng-Chi, C., and L. Wen-Hsiung. "Genomic Divergences between Humans and Other Hominoids and the Effective Population Size of the Common Ancestor of Humans and Chimpanzees." *Am J Hum Genet* 68:2 (2001): 444–456.

19. Gigerenzer, G. *Calculated Risks.* New York, NY: Simon & Schuster, 2002.

20. Surowiecki, J. *The Wisdom of Crowds.* New York, NY: Doubleday, 2004.

21. Hickey, S., and H. Roberts. *Ascorbate: The Science of Vitamin C.* Lulu Press, 2004.

22. Ibid.

23. Stephen, R., and T. Utecht. "Scurvy Identified in the Emergency Department: A Case Report." *J Emerg Med* 21:3 (2001): 235–237. Weinstein, M., P. Babyn, S. Zlotkin. "An Orange a Day Keeps the Doctor Away: Scurvy in the Year." *Pediatrics* 108:3 (2001): E55.

24. Enstrom, J.E., L.E. Kanim, M.A. Klein. "Vitamin C Intake and Mortality

among a Sample of the United States Population." *Epidemiology* 3:3 (1992): 194–202.

25. Enstrom, J.E. "Counterpoint—Vitamin C and Mortality." *Nutr Today* 28 (1993): 28–32.

26. Knekt, P., J. Ritz, M.A. Pereira, et al. "Antioxidant Vitamins and Coronary Heart Disease Risk: A Pooled Analysis of 9 Cohorts." *Am J Clin Nutr* 80:6 (2004): 1508–1520.

27. Osganian, S.K., M.J. Stampfer. E. Rimm, et al. "Vitamin C and Risk of Coronary Heart Disease in Women." *J Am Coll Cardiol* 42:2 (2003): 246–252.

28. Yokoyama, T., C. Date, Y. Kokubo, et al. "Serum Vitamin C Concentration was Inversely Associated with Subsequent 20-year Incidence of Stroke in a Japanese Rural Community: The Shibata Study." *Stroke* 31:10 (2000): 2287–2294.

29. Kushi, L.H., A.R. Folsom, R.J. Prineas, et al. "Dietary Antioxidant Vitamins and Death from Coronary Heart Disease in Postmenopausal Women." *N Engl J Med* 334:18 (1996): 1156–1162. Losonczy, K.G., T.B. Harris, R.J. Havlik. "Vitamin E and Vitamin C Supplement Use and Risk of All-cause and Coronary Heart Disease Mortality in Older Persons: The Established Populations for Epidemiologic Studies of the Elderly." *Am J Clin Nutr* 64:2 (1996): 190–196.

30. Frei, B. "To C or Not to C, That is the Question!" *J Am Coll Cardiol* 42:2 (2003): 253–255.

31. Steinmetz, K.A., and J.D. Potter. "Vegetables, Fruit, and Cancer Prevention: A Review." *J Am Diet Assoc* 96:10 (1996): 1027–1039.

32. Kromhout, D. "Essential Micronutrients in Relation to Carcinogenesis." *Am J Clin Nutr* 45:5 Suppl (1987): 1361–1367.

33. Feiz, H.R., and S. Mobarhan. "Does Vitamin C Intake Slow the Progression of Gastric Cancer in *Helicobacter pylori*–infected Populations?" *Nutr Rev* 60:1 (2002): 34–36.

34. Michels, K.B., L. Holmberg, L. Bergkvist, et al. "Dietary Antioxidant Vitamins, Retinol, and Breast Cancer Incidence in a Cohort of Swedish Women." *Intl J Cancer* 91:4 (2001): 563–567.

35. Zhang, S., D.J. Hunter, M.R. Forman, et al. "Dietary Carotenoids and Vitamins A, C, and E and Risk of Breast Cancer." *J Natl Cancer Inst* 91:6 (1999): 547–556.

36. Hoffer, A. *Adventures in Psychiatry: The Scientific Memoirs of Dr. Abram Hoffer.* Caledon, Ontario, Canada: Kos Publishing, 2005.

37. Greensfelder, L. "Infectious Diseases: Polio Outbreak Raises Questions about Vaccine." *Science* 290:5498 (2000): 1867b–1869b. Martin, J. "Vaccine-derived Poliovirus from Long-term Excretors and the End Game of Polio Eradication." *Biologicals* 34:2 (2006): 117–122.

38. Ermatinger, J.W. *Decline and Fall of the Roman Empire.* Westport, CT: Greenwood Press, 2004.

39. Watanabe, C., and H. Satoh. "Evolution of Our Understanding of Methylmercury as a Health Threat." *Environ Health Perspect* 104:Suppl 2 (1996): 367–379. Mortada, W.L., M.A. Sobh, M.M. El-Defrawy, et al. "Mercury in Dental Restoration: Is There a Risk of Nephrotoxicity?" *J Nephrol* 15:2 (2002): 171–176.

40. Cheng, Y., W.C. Willett, J. Schwartz, et al. "Relation of Nutrition to Bone Lead and Blood Lead Levels in Middle-aged to Elderly Men, The Normative Aging Study." *Am J Epidemiol* 147:12 (1998): 1162–1174.

41. Simon, J.A., and E.S. Hudes. "Relationship of Ascorbic Acid to Blood Lead Levels." *JAMA* 281:24 (1999): 2289–2293.

42. Dawson, E.B., D.R. Evans, W.A. Harris, et al. "The Effect of Ascorbic Acid Supplementation on the Blood Lead Levels of Smokers." *J Am Coll Nutr* 18:2 (1999): 166–170.

43. Jacques, P.F. "The Potential Preventive Effects of Vitamins for Cataract and Age-related Macular Degeneration." *Intl J Vitamin Nutr Res* 69:3 (1999): 198–205.

44. Simon, J.A., and E.S. Hudes. "Serum Ascorbic Acid and Other Correlates of Self-reported Cataract among Older Americans." *J Clin Epidemiol* 52:12 (1999): 1207–1211.

45. Jacques, P.F., L.T. Chylack, S.E. Hankinson, et al. "Long-term Nutrient Intake and Early Age-related Nuclear Lens Opacities." *Arch Ophthalmol* 119:7 (2001): 1009–1019.

46. Age-Related Eye Disease Study Research Group. "A Randomized, Placebo-controlled, Clinical Trial of High-dose Supplementation with Vitamins C and E and Beta Carotene for Age-related Cataract and Vision Loss: AREDS Report No. 9." *Arch Ophthalmol* 119:10 (2001): 1439–1452.

Chapter 2: The Pioneers of Vitamin C Research

1. Cott, A. "Irwin Stone: A Tribute." *Orthomolecular Psych* 14 (2nd Quarter 1985): 150.

2. Stone, I. "On the Genetic Etiology of Scurvy." *Acta Genet Med Gemellol* 15 (1966): 345–350.

3. Stone, I. "The Genetic Disease, Hypoascorbemia: A Fresh Approach to an Ancient Disease and Some of Its Medical Implications." *Acta Genet Med Gemellol* 16:1 (1967): 52–62. Stone, I. "Humans, the Mammalian Mutants." *Am Lab* 6:4 (1974): 32–39.

4. Stone, I. "Eight Decades of Scurvy: The Case History of a Misleading Dietary Hypothesis." *Orthomolecular Psych* 8:2 (1979): 58–62.

5. Stone, I. "Sudden Death. A Look Back from Ascorbate's 50th Anniversary." *Australas Nurses J* 8:9 (1979): 9–13, 39.

6. Kalokerinos, A. *Every Second Child*. Melbourne, Australia: Thomas Nelson (Australia) Ltd., 1974.

7. Stone, I. "Hypoascorbemia, Our Most Widespread Disease." *Natl Health Fed Bull* 18:10 (1972): 6–9.

8. Stone, I. "The Natural History of Ascorbic Acid in the Evolution of the Mammals and Primates and Its Significance for Present Day Man." *J Orthomolecular Psych* 1:2–3 (1972): 82–89.

9. Stone, I. "Megadoses of Vitamin C." *Nutr Today* 10:3 (1975): 35.

10. Rimland, B. "In Memoriam: Irwin Stone 1907–1984." *J Orthomolecular Psych* 13:4 (1984): 285.

11. Hoffer, A. "The Vitamin Paradigm Wars." *Townsend Letter for Doctors and Patients* 155 (1996): 56–60. Available online at: http://www.doctoryourself.com/hoffer_paradigm.html.

12. Stone, I. "Hypoascorbemia: The Genetic Disease Causing the Human Requirement for Exogenous Ascorbic Acid." *Perspect Biol Med* 10 (1966): 133–134

13. Nathens, A.B., M.J. Neff, G.J. Jurkovich, et al. "Randomized, Prospective Trial of Antioxidant Supplementation in Critically Ill Surgical Patients." *Ann Surg* 236:6 (2002): 814–822.

14. Stone, I. "Fifty Years of Research on Ascorbate and the Genetics of Scurvy." *Orthomolecular Psych* 13:4 (1984): 280.

15. Related to Andrew Saul. *Doctor Yourself Newsletter* 4:23 (November 2004).

16. Stone, I. "Letter to Albert Szent-Gyorgyi." National Foundation for Cancer Research, Woods Hole, Massachusetts, August 30, 1982.

17. Stone, I. "Cancer Therapy in the Light of the Natural History of Ascorbic Acid." *J Intl Acad Metabol* 3:1 (1974): 56–61. Stone, I. "The Genetics of Scurvy and the Cancer Problem." *J Orthomolecular Psych* 5:3 (1976): 183–190. Stone,

I. "The Possible Role of Mega-ascorbate in the Endogenous Synthesis of Interferon." *Med Hypotheses* 6:3 (March 1980): 309–314. Stone, I. "Inexpensive Interferon Therapy of Cancer and the Viral Diseases Now." *Australas Nurses J* 10:3 (March 1981): 25–28.

18. Cathcart, R.F. "Vitamin C, Titration to Bowel Tolerance, Anascorbemia, and Acute Induced Scurvy." *Med Hypothesis* 7 (1981): 1359–1376. Available online at: http://www.doctoryour self.com/titration.html.

19. Levine, M., C. Conry-Cantilena, Y. Wang, et al. "Vitamin C Pharmacokinetics in Healthy Volunteers: Evidence for a Recommended Dietary Allowance." *Proc Natl Acad Sci USA* 93 (1996): 3704–3709. Levine, M., Y. Wang, S.J. Padayatty, et al. (2001) "A New Recommended Dietary Allowance of Vitamin C for Healthy Young Women." *Proc Natl Acad Sci USA* 98:17 (2001): 9842–9846.

20. Hickey, S., and H. Roberts. *Ridiculous Dietary Allowance*. Lulu Press, 2004.

21. Smith, L. *Vitamin C as a Fundamental Medicine*. (Re-titled *Clinical Guide to the Use of Vitamin C: The Clinical Experiences of Frederick R. Klenner M.D.*) Tacoma, WA: Life Sciences Press, 1991.

22. Levy, T.E. *Vitamin C, Infectious Diseases, and Toxins: Curing the Incurable*. Xlibris, 2002.

23. Miller, F. "Dr. Klenner Urges Taking Vitamins in Huge Doses." *Greensboro Daily News* (December 13, 1977): A8–A10.

24. Kalokerinos, A. *Every Second Child*. Melbourne, Australia: Thomas Nelson, 1974.

25. Pauling, L. In Stone, I. *Vitamin C as a Fundamental Medicine: Abstracts of Dr. Frederick R. Klenner, M.D.'s Published and Unpublished Work*. (Re-titled *Clinical Guide to the Use of Vitamin C: The Clinical Experiences of Frederick R. Klenner M.D.*) Tacoma, WA: Life Sciences Press, 1991.

26. Smith, L. *Feed Yourself Right*. New York, NY: Dell, 1983.

27. Smith, Lendon H., and Joseph G. Hattersley. "Victory Over Crib Death." (June 2000.) Mercola.com. Available online at: http://www.mercola.com/2000/nov/5/victory_over_sids.htm.

28. Lendon Smith's former website: www.Smithsez.com.

29. "Vaccine-derived Polioviruses—Update." *Wkly Epidemiol Record* 81:42 (2006): 398–404. Tebbens, R.J., M.A. Pallansch, O.M. Kew, et al. "Risks of Paralytic Disease Due to Wild or Vaccine-derived Poliovirus after Eradication." *Risk Anal* 26:6 (2006): 1471–1505. Jenkins, P.C., and J.F. Modlin. "Decision

Analysis in Planning for a Polio Outbreak in the United States." *Pediatrics* 118:2 (2006): 611–618. Friedrich, F. "Molecular Evolution of Oral Poliovirus Vaccine Strains during Multiplication in Humans and Possible Implications for Global Eradication of Poliovirus." *Acta Virol* 44:2 (2000): 109–117.

30. Miller, N.Z.. "Vaccines and Natural Health." *Mothering* (Spring 1994): 44–54.

31. Advisory Committee on Immunization Practices. "Notice to Readers: Recommended Childhood Immunization Schedule—United States." *MMWR Weekly Rep* 49:2 (January 2000): 35–38.

32. Jungeblut, C.W. "Inactivation of Poliomyelitis Virus by Crystalline Vitamin C (Ascorbic Acid)." *J Exp Med* 62 (1935): 317–321.

33. Jungeblut, C.W., and R.L. Zwemer. "Inactivation of Diphtheria Toxin in Vivo and in Vitro by Crystalline Vitamin C (Ascorbic Acid)." *Proc Soc Exp Biol Med* 32 (1935): 1229–1234. Jungeblut, C.W. "Inactivation of Tetanus Toxin by Crystalline Vitamin C (L-Ascorbic Acid)." *J Immunol* 33 (1937): 203–214.

34. Ely, J.T.A. "A Unity of Science, Especially among Physicists, is Urgently Needed to End Medicine's Lethal Misdirection." ArXiv.org, Cornell University Library (March 2004). Available online at: http://arxive.org/abs/physics/0403023.

35. "Polio Clues." *Time Magazine* (September 18, 1939).

36. Klenner, F.R. "The Use of Vitamin C as an Antibiotic." *J Appl Nutr* 6 (1953): 274–278.

37. Hickey, S., and H. Roberts. *Ascorbate: The Science of Vitamin C.* Lulu Press, 2004.

38. Stone, I. "Viral Infection." *The Healing Factor,* Chapter 13. New York, NY: Grosset and Dunlap, 1972.

39. Landwehr, R. "The Origin of the 42-Year Stonewall of Vitamin C." *J Orthomolecular Med* 6:2 (1991): 99–103.

40. Klenner, F.R. "The Treatment of Poliomyelitis and Other Virus Diseases with Vitamin C." *Southern Med Surg* (July 1949): 209.

41. Chan, D., S.R. Lamande, W.G. Cole, et al. "Regulation of Procollagen Synthesis and Processing during Ascorbate-induced Extracellular Matrix Accumulation in Vitro." *Biochem J* 269:1 (1990): 175–181. Franceschi, R.T., B.S. Iyer, Y. Cui. "Effects of Ascorbic Acid on Collagen Matrix Formation and Osteoblast Differentiation in Murine MC3T3-E1 Cells." *J Bone Miner Res* 9:6 (1994): 843–854.

42. McCormick, W.J. "The Striae of Pregnancy: A New Etiological Concept." *Med Record* (August 1948).

43. Stone, I. "The Genetic Disease, Hypoascorbemia: A Fresh Approach to an Ancient Disease and Some of Its Medical Implications." *Acta Genet Med Gemellol* 16:1 (1967): 52–60.

44. McCormick, W.J. "Have We Forgotten the Lesson of Scurvy?" *J Appl Nutr* 15:1–2 (1962): 4–12.

45. McCormick, W.J. "Cancer: The Preconditioning Factor in Pathogenesis." *Arch Pediatr NY* 71 (1954): 313. McCormick, W.J. "Cancer: A Collagen Disease, Secondary to a Nutritional Deficiency?" *Arch Pediatr* 76 (1959): 166.

46. Pincus, F. "Acute Lymphatic Leukaemia." In *Nothnagel's Encyclopedia of Practical Medicine,* American Ed. Philadelphia, PA: W.B. Saunders, 1905, pp. 552–574.

47. Gonzalez, M.J., J.R. Miranda-Massari, E.M. Mora, et al. "Orthomolecular Oncology: A Mechanistic View of Intravenous Ascorbate's Chemotherapeutic Activity." *P R Health Sci J* 21:1 (March 2002): 39–41. Hickey, S., and H. Roberts. *Cancer: Nutrition and Survival.* Lulu Press, 2005.

48. McCormick, W.J. "Coronary Thrombosis: A New Concept of Mechanism and Etiology." *Clin Med* 4:7 (July 1957).

49. Scannapieco, F.A., and R.J. Genco. "Association of Periodontal Infections with Atherosclerotic and Pulmonary Diseases." *J Periodontal Res* 34:7 (1999): 340–345.

50. Paterson, J.C. "Some Factors in the Causation of Intimal Hemorrhage and in the Precipitation of Coronary Thrombosis." *Can Med Assoc J* 44 (1941): 114.

51. Enstrom, J.E., L.E. Kanim, M.A. Klein. "Vitamin C Intake and Mortality among a Sample of the United States Population." *Epidemiology* 3:3 (1992): 194–202.

52. McCormick, W.J. "The Changing Incidence and Mortality of Infectious Disease in Relation to Changed Trends in Nutrition." *Med Record* (September 1947).

53. McCormick, W.J. "Ascorbic Acid as a Chemotherapeutic Agent." *Arch Pediatr NY* 69 (1952): 151–155. Available online at: http://www.doctoryourself.com/mccormick1951.html.

54. Curhan, G.C., W.C. Willett, F.E. Speizer, et al. "Intake of Vitamins B$_6$ and C and the Risk of Kidney Stones in Women." *J Am Soc Nephrol* 10:4 (1999): 840–845.

55. McCormick, W.J. "Lithogenesis and Hypovitaminosis." *Med Record* 159:7 (1946): 410–413.

56. McCormick, W.J. "Intervertebral Disc Lesions: A New Etiological Concept." *Arch Pediatr NY* 71 (1954): 29–33.

57. Salomon, L.L., and D.W. Stubbs. "Some Aspects of the Metabolism of Ascorbic Acid in Rats." *Ann NY Acad Sci* 92 (1961): 128–140. Conney, A.H., et al. "Metabolic Interactions between L-Ascorbic Acid and Drugs." *Ann NY Acad Sci* 92 (1961): 115–127.

58. Armour, J., K. Tyml, D. Lidington, et al. "Ascorbate Prevents Microvascular Dysfunction in the Skeletal Muscle of the Septic Rat." *J Appl Physiol* 90:3 (2001): 795–803.

59. Conney, A.H., C.A. Bray, C. Evans, et al. "Metabolic Interactions between L-Ascorbic Acid and Drugs." *Ann NY Acad Sci* 92 (1961): 115–127.

60. Pauling, L. "Evolution and the Need for Ascorbic Acid." *Proc Natl Acad Sci USA* 67 (1970): 1643–1648.

61. Hickey, S., and H. Roberts. *Ridiculous Dietary Allowance*. Lulu Press, 2005.

Chapter 3: Taking Vitamin C

1. Hickey, S., and H. Roberts. *Ridiculous Dietary Allowance*. Lulu Press, 2005.

2. Ibid.

3. Expert Group on Vitamins and Minerals. "Review of Vitamin C." U.K. Government Update Paper EVM/99/21/P. London: Expert Group on Vitamins and Minerals, November 1999.

4. McCormick, W.J. "Coronary Thrombosis: A New Concept of Mechanism and Etiology." *Clin Med* 4:7 (July 1957) 839–845.

5. Levine, M., C. Conry-Cantilena, Y. Wang, et al. "Vitamin C Pharmacokinetics in Healthy Volunteers: Evidence for a Recommended Dietary Allowance." *Proc Natl Acad Sci USA* 93 (1996): 3704–3709. Standing Committee on Dietary Reference Intakes, Institute of Medicine. *Dietary Reference Intakes for Vitamin C, Vitamin E, Selenium, and Carotenoids: A Report of the Panel on Dietary Antioxidants and Related Compounds*. Washington, DC: National Academy Press, 2000. Levine, M., Y. Wang, S.J. Padayatty, et al. "A New Recommended Dietary Allowance of Vitamin C for Healthy Young Women." *Proc Natl Acad Sci USA* 98:17 (2001): 9842–9846.

6. Kallner, A., I. Hartmann, D. Hornig. "Steady-state Turnover and Body Pool of Ascorbic Acid in Man." *Am J Clin Nutr* 32 (1979): 530–539.

7. Baker, E.M., R.E. Hodges, J. Hood, et al. "Metabolism of Ascorbic-1-14C Acid in Experimental Human Scurvy." *Am J Clin Nutr* 22:5 (1969): 549–558.

8. Kallner, A., I. Hartmann, D. Hornig. "On the Absorption of Ascorbic Acid in Man." *Intl J Vitamin Nutr Res* 47 (1977): 383–388. Hornig, D.H., and U. Moser. "The Safety of High Vitamin C Intakes in Man." In Counsell, J.N., and D.H. Hornig (eds.). *Vitamin C (Ascorbic Acid)*. London: Applied Science Publishers, 1981, pp. 225–248.

9. Young, V.R. "Evidence for a Recommended Dietary Allowance for Vitamin C from Pharmacokinetics: A Comment and Analysis." *Proc Natl Acad Sci USA* 93 (1996): 14344–14348. Ginter, E. "Current Views of the Optimum Dose of Vitamin C." *Slovakofarma Rev* XII (2002): 1, 4–8.

10. Hornig, D. "Distribution of Ascorbic Acid, Metabolites and Analogues in Man and Animals." *Ann NY Acad Sci* 258 (1975): 103–118. Moser, U. "The Uptake of Ascorbic Acid by Leukocytes." *Ann NY Acad Sci* 198 (1987): 200–215.

11. Watson, R.W.G "Redox Regulation of Neutrophil Apoptosis, Antioxidants and Redox Signalling." *Forum Rev* 4:1 (2002): 97–104. Kinnula, V.L., Y. Soini, K. Kvist-Makela, et al. "Antioxidant Defense Mechanisms in Human Neutrophils, Antioxidants and Redox Signalling." *Forum Rev* 4:1 (2002): 27–34.

12. Hickey, S., and H. Roberts. *Ascorbate: The Science of Vitamin C*. Lulu Press, 2004.

13. Washko, P., and M.J. Levine. "Inhibition of Ascorbic Acid Transport in Human Neutrophils by Glucose." *Biol Chem* 267:33 (1992): 23568–23574.

14. Santisteban, G.A., and J.T. Ely. "Glycemic Modulation of Tumor Tolerance in a Mouse Model of Breast Cancer." *Biochem Biophys Res Commun* 132:3 (1985): 1174–1179. Hamel, E.E., G.A. Santisteban, J.T. Ely, et al. "Hyperglycemia and Reproductive Defects in Non-diabetic Gravidas: A Mouse Model Test of a New Theory." *Life Sci* 39:16 (1986): 1425–1428. Ely, J.T. "Glycemic Modulation of Tumor Tolerance." *J Orthomolecular Med* 11:1 (1996): 23–34. Fladeby, C., R. Skar, G. Serck-Hanssen. "Distinct Regulation of Glucose Transport and GLUT1/GLUT3 Transporters by Glucose Deprivation and IGF-I in Chromaffin Cells." *Biochim Biophys Acta* 1593:2–3 (2003): 201–208.

15. Daruwala, R., J. Song, W.S. Koh, et al. "Cloning and Functional Characterization of the Human Sodium-dependent Vitamin C Transporters hSVCT1 and hSVCT2." *FEBS Lett* 460:3 (1999): 480–484. Tsukaguchi, H., T. Tokui, B. Mackenzie, et al. "A Family of Mammalian Na+-dependent L-Ascorbic Acid Transporters." *Nature* 399 (1999): 70–75.

16. Olson, A.L., and J.E. Pessin. "Structure, Function and Regulation of the Mammalian Facilitative Glucose Transporter Gene Family." *Annu Rev Nutr* 16 (1996): 235–256. Mueckler, M. "Facilitative Glucose Transporters." *Eur J Biochem* 219 (1994): 713–725.

17. Cathcart, R.F. "Vitamin C: The Nontoxic, Nonrate-limited, Antioxidant Free Radical Scavenger." *Med Hypotheses* 18 (1985): 61–77.

18. Douglas, R.M., H. Hemila, R. D'Souza, et al. "Vitamin C for Preventing and Treating the Common Cold." *Cochrane Database Syst Rev* 18:4 (2004): CD000980.

19. Drisco, J. Data presented at the Nutritional Medicine Today Conference, Toronto, Canada, 2007.

20. Yung, S., M. Mayersohn, J.B. Robinson. "Ascorbic Acid Absorption in Humans: A Comparison among Several Dosage Forms." *J Pharm Sci* 71:3 (1982): 282–285.

21. Gregory, J.F. "Ascorbic Acid Bioavailability in Foods and Supplements." *Nutr Rev* 51:10 (1993): 301–303.

22. Pelletier, O., and M.O. Keith. "Bioavailability of Synthetic and Natural Ascorbic Acid." *J Am Diet Assoc* 64 (1964): 271–275.

23. Mangels, A.R., G. Block, C.M. Frey, et al. "The Bioavailability to Humans of Ascorbic Acid from Oranges, Orange Juice and Cooked Broccoli is Similar to that of Synthetic Ascorbic Acid." *J Nutr* 123:6 (1993): 1054–1061.

24. Gregory, J.F. "Ascorbic Acid Bioavailability in Foods and Supplements." *Nutr Rev* 51:10 (1993): 301–303.

25. Vinson, J.A., and P. Bose. "Comparative Bioavailability to Humans of Ascorbic Acid Alone or in a Citrus Extract." *Am J Clin Nutr* 48:3 (1988): 601–604. Johnston, C.S., and B. Luo. "Comparison of the Absorption and Excretion of Three Commercially Available Sources of Vitamin C." *J Am Diet Assoc* 94:7 (1994): 779–781.

26. Spiclin, P., M. Gasperlin, V. Kmetec. "Stability of Ascorbyl Palmitate in Topical Microemulsions." *Intl J Pharm* 222:2 (2001): 271–279.

27. De Ritter, E., N. Cohen, S.H. Rubin. "Physiological Availability of Dehydro-L-Ascorbic Acid and Palmitoyl-L-Ascorbic Acid." *Science* 113:2944 (1951): 628–631.

28. Levine, M., S.C. Rumsey, R. Daruwala, et al. "Criteria and Recommendations for Vitamin C Intake." *JAMA* 281 (1999): 1415–1423.

29. American Association of Poison Control Centers (AAPCC). "Annual Report of the American Association of Poison Control Centers' National Poisoning and Exposure Database." (Formerly known as the Toxic Exposure Surveillance System.) Washington, DC: AAPCC, 1983–2005.

30. National Center for Health Statistics (NCHS). "1987 Summary: National Hospital Discharge Survey." Washington, DC: NCHS, 1987.

31. Ray, W.A., M.R. Griffin, R.I. Shorr. "Adverse Drug Reactions and the Elderly." *Health Affairs* 9 (1990): 114–122.

32. Ostapowicz, G., R.J. Fontana, F.V. Schiødt, et al. "Results of a Prospective Study of Acute Liver Failure at 17 Tertiary Care Centers in the United States." *Ann Intern Med* 137 (2002): 947–954.

33. Nourjah, P., S.R. Ahmad, C. Karwoski, et al. "Estimates of Acetaminophen (Paracetomal)-associated Overdoses in the United States." *Pharmacoepidemiol Drug Safety* 15:6 (2006): 398–405.

34. Gurkirpal, S. "Recent Considerations in Nonsteroidal Anti-inflammatory Drug Gastropathy." *Am J Med* (July 1998): 31S. Wolfe, M., D. Lichtenstein, S. Gurkirpal. "Gastrointestinal Toxicity of Nonsteroidal Anti-inflammatory Drugs." *N Engl J Med* 340:24 (1999): 1888–1889.

35. Kohn, L., J. Corrigan, M. Donaldson. *To Err is Human: Building a Safer Health System.* Washington, DC: National Academy Press, 1999.

36. Leape, L.L. "Unnecessary Surgery." *Annu Rev Public Health* 13 (1992): 363–383. Phillips, D.P., N. Christenfeld, L.M. Glynn. "Increase in U.S. Medication-error Deaths between 1983 and 1993." *Lancet* 351:9103 (1998): 643–644. Lazarou, J., B.H. Pomeranz, P.N. Corey. "Incidence of Adverse Drug Reactions in Hospitalized Patients: A Meta-analysis of Prospective Studies." *JAMA* 279:15 (April 1998): 1200–1205.

37. Johnston, C.S. "Biomarkers for Establishing a Tolerable Upper Intake Level for Vitamin C." *Nutr Rev* 57 (1999): 71–77. Garewal, H.S., and A.T. Diplock. "How 'Safe' are Antioxidant Vitamins?" *Drug Safety* 13:1 (July 1995): 8–14. Diplock, A.T. "Safety of Antioxidant Vitamins and Beta-carotene." *Am J Clin Nutr* 62:6 Suppl (1995): 1510S–1516S.

38. McCormick, W.J. "Lithogenesis and Hypovitaminosis." *Med Record* 159 (1946): 410–413.

39. van Aswegen, C.H., J.C. Dirksen van Sckalckwyk, P.J. du Toit, et al. "The Effect of Calcium and Magnesium Ions on Urinary Urokinase and Sialidase Activity." *Urol Res* 20:1 (1992): 41–44.

40. Lemann Jr., J., W.F. Piering, E. Lennon. "Possible Role of Carbohydrate-induced Calciuria in Calcium Oxalate Kidney-stone Formation." *N Engl J Med* 280:5 (1969): 232–237.

41. Chalmers, A.H, D.M. Cowley, J.M. Brown. "A Possible Etiological Role for Ascorbate in Calculi Formation." *Clin Chem* 32:2 (1986): 333–336. Baxmann, A.C., G. De O, C. Mendonça, et al. "Effect of Vitamin C Supplements on Urinary Oxalate and pH in Calcium Stone-forming Patients." *Kidney Intl* 63 (2003): 1066–1071. Auer, B.L., D. Auer, A.L. Rodgers. "The Effect of Ascor-

bic Acid Ingestion on the Biochemical and Physicochemical Risk Factors Associated with Calcium Oxalate Kidney Stone Formation." *Clin Chem Lab Med* 36:3 (1998): 143–147.

42. Tiselius, H. "Stone Incidence and Prevention." *Brazil J Urol* 26:5 (2000): 452–462.

43. Curhan, G.C., W.C. Willett, F.E. Speizer, et al. "Megadose Vitamin C Consumption Does Not Cause Kidney Stones. Intake of Vitamins B_6 and C and the Risk of Kidney Stones in Women." *J Am Soc Nephrol* 4 (April 1999): 840–845.

44. Curhan, G.C., W.C. Willett, E.B. Rimm, et al. "A Prospective Study of the Intake of Vitamins C and B_6, and the Risk of Kidney Stones in Men." *J Urol* 155:6 (1996): 1847–1851.

45. Ruwende, C., and A. Hill. "Glucose-6-phosphate Dehydrogenase Deficiency and Malaria." *J Mol Med* 76:8 (1998): 581–588.

46. Liu, T.Z., T.F. Lin, I.J. Hung, et al. "Enhanced Susceptibility of Erythrocytes Deficient in Glucose-6-phosphate Dehydrogenase to Alloxan/glutathione-induced Decrease in Red Cell Deformability." *Life Sci* 55:3 (1994): 55–60.

47. Ballin, A., E.J. Brown, G. Koren, et al. "Vitamin C-induced Erythrocyte Damage in Premature Infants." *J Pediatr* 113 (1998): 114–120. Mentzer, W.C., and E. Collier. "Hydrops Fetalis Associated with Erythrocyte G-6-PD Deficiency and Maternal Ingestion of Fava Beans and Ascorbic Acid." *J Pediatr* 86 (1975): 565–567. Campbell Jr., G.D., M.H. Steinberg, J.D. Bower. "Ascorbic Acid–induced Hemolysis in G-6-PD Deficiency." *Ann Intern Med* 82 (1975): 810. Rees, D.C., H. Kelsey, J.D.M. Richards. "Acute Hemolysis Induced by High-dose Ascorbic Acid in Glucose-6-phosphate Dehydrogenase Deficiency." *Br Med J* 306 (1993): 841–842.

48. Council for Responsible Nutrition. "Fact Sheet: Are Vitamins and Minerals Safe for Persons with G6PD Deficiency?" Washington, DC: Council for Responsible Nutrition, 2005. Available online at: http://www.crnusa.org/pdfs/CRN_G6PDDeficiency_0305.pdf.

49. Cook, J.D., S.S. Watson, K.M. Simpson, et al. "The Effect of High Ascorbic Acid Supplementation on Body Iron Stores." *Blood* 64 (1984): 721–726. Hunt, J.R., S.K. Gallagher, L.K. Johnson. "Effect of Ascorbic Acid on Apparent Iron Absorption by Women with Low Iron Stores." *Am J Clin Nutr* 59 (1994): 1381–1385.

50. Bacon, B.R., J.K. Olynyk, E.M. Brunt, et al. "HFE Genotype in Patients with Hemochromatosis and Other Liver Diseases." *Ann Intern Med* 130 (1999): 953–962.

51. McLaran, C.J., J.H.N. Bett, J.A. Nye, et al. "Congestive Cardiomyopathy

and Haemochromatosis—Rapid Progression Possibly Accelerated by Excessive Ingestion of Ascorbic Acid." *Aust NZ J Med* 12 (1982): 187–188.

52. Berger, T.M., M.C. Polidori, A. Dabbagh, et al. "Antioxidant Activity of Vitamin C in Iron-overloaded Human Plasma." *J Biol Chem* 272 (1997): 15656–15660.

53. Cathcart, R.F. Personal communication, 2006.

54. Appell, D. "The New Uncertainty Principle: For Complex Environmental Issues, Science Learns to Take a Backseat to Political Precaution." *Sci Am* (January 2001). Available online at: http://www.sciam.com/article.cfm?colID=18& articleID=000C3111-2859-1C71-84A9809EC588EF21.

Chapter 4: Conventional Medicine versus Vitamin C

1. Lanfranchi, A. "The Abortion-Breast Cancer Link: What Today's Evidence Shows." *Ethics and Medics* 28:1 (January 2003): 1–4.

2. Lemjabbar, H., D. Li, M. Gallup, et al. "Tobacco Smoke-induced Lung Cell Proliferation Mediated by Tumor Necrosis Factor Alpha–converting Enzyme and Amphiregulin." *J Biol Chem* 278:28 (2003): 26202–26207.

3. Bernert, J.T., R.B. Jain, J.L. Pirkle, et al. "Urinary Tobacco-specific Nitrosamines and 4-Aminobiphenyl Hemoglobin Adducts Measured in Smokers of Either Regular or Light Cigarettes." *Nicotine Tobacco Res* 7:5 (2005): 729–738.

4. Zhou, H., G.M. Calaf, T.K. Hei. "Malignant Transformation of Human Bronchial Epithelial Cells with the Tobacco-specific Nitrosamine, 4-(Methylnitrosamino)-1-(3-pyridyl)-1-butanone." *Intl J Cancer* 106:6 (2003): 821–826. Rubin, H. "Selective Clonal Expansion and Microenvironmental Permissiveness in Tobacco Carcinogenesis." *Oncogene* 21:48 (2002): 7392–7411.

5. D'Agostini, F., R.M. Balansky, C. Bennicelli, et al. (2001) "Pilot Studies Evaluating the Lung Tumor Yield in Cigarette Smoke-exposed Mice." *Intl J Oncol* 18:3 (2001): 607–615. Coggins, C.R. "A Minireview of Chronic Animal Inhalation Studies with Mainstream Cigarette Smoke." *Inhal Toxicol* 14:10 (2002): 991–1002.

6. Witschi, H., I. Espiritu, M. Ly, et al. "The Chemopreventive Effects of Orally Administered Dexamethasone in Strain A/J Mice Following Cessation of Smoke Exposure." *Inhal Toxicol* 17:2 (2005): 119–122. Curtin, G.M., M.A. Higuchi, P.H. Ayres, et al. "Lung Tumorigenicity in A/J and rasH2 Transgenic Mice Following Mainstream Tobacco Smoke Inhalation." *Toxicol Sci* 81:1 (2004): 26–34. Witschi, H. "Induction of Lung Cancer by Passive Smoking in an Animal Model System." *Methods Mol Med* 74 (2003): 441–455.

7. Epstein, S. *Stop Cancer Before It Starts Campaign: How to Win the Losing War on Cancer.* Chicago, IL: Cancer Prevention Coalition, 2003. Doll, R., and R. Peto. "The Causes of Cancer: Quantitative Estimates of Avoidable Risks of Cancer in the U.S. Today." *J Natl Cancer Inst* 66 (1981): 1191–1308. Castleman, B. "Doll's 1955 Study on Cancer from Asbestos." *Am J Ind Med* 39 (2001): 237–240. Doll, R. "Effects of Exposure to Vinyl Chloride and Assessment of the Evidence." *Scand J Work Environ Health* 14 (1988): 61–78.

8. An appreciation of Bradford Hill from Professor Peter Armitage, former president of the Royal Statistical Society. *J Royal Stat Soc* 154:3 (1991):482–484

9. Proctor, R.N. *Nazi War on Cancer.* Princeton, NJ: Princeton University Press, 2000.

10. Doll, R., et al. "Mortality in Relation to Smoking: Forty Years' Observations on Male British Doctors." *Br Med J* 309 (1994): 901–909. Sharp, D. "Cancer Prevention Tomorrow." *Lancet* 341 (1993): 486.

11. MacMahon, B., S. Yen, D. Trichopoulos, et al. "Coffee and Cancer of the Pancreas." *N Engl J Med* 304:11 (1981): 630–633.

12. Weinstein, N.D. "Reactions to Life-style Warnings: Coffee and Cancer." *Health Educ Q* 12:2 (1985): 129–134. Tavani, A., and C. La Vecchia. "Coffee and Cancer: A Review of Epidemiological Studies, 1990–1999." *Eur J Cancer Prev* 9:4 (2000): 241–256.

13. Kurozawa, Y., I. Ogimoto, A. Shibata, et al. "Coffee and Risk of Death from Hepatocellular Carcinoma in a Large Cohort Study in Japan." *Br J Cancer* 93:5 (2005): 607–610. Shimazu, T., Y. Tsubono, S. Kuriyama, et al. "Coffee Consumption and the Risk of Primary Liver Cancer: Pooled Analysis of Two Prospective Studies in Japan." *Intl J Cancer* 116:1 (2005): 150–154. Jordan, S.J., D.M. Purdie, A.C. Green, et al. "Coffee, Tea and Caffeine and Risk of Epithelial Ovarian Cancer." *Cancer Causes Control* 15:4 (2004): 359–365. Jacobsen, B.K., E. Bjelke, G. Kvale, et al. "Coffee Drinking, Mortality, and Cancer Incidence: Results from a Norwegian Prospective Study." *J Natl Cancer Inst* 76:5 (1986): 823–831.

14. Breslow, N.E., and N.E. Day. *Statistical Methods in Cancer Research, Vol. 1 and 2: The Analysis of Case-Control Studies.* Lyons, France: International Agency for Research on Cancer, 1980. Rothman, K.J., and S. Greenland. *Modern Epidemiology.* Boston, MA: Lippincott-Raven, 1998. Grimes, D., and K.F. Schulz. "Epidemiology Series." *Lancet* 359 (2002): 57–61, 145–149, 248–252, 341–345, 431–434. Pocock, S.J., T.J. Collier, K.J. Dandreo, et al. "Issues in the Reporting of Epidemiological Studies: A Survey of Recent Practice." *Br Med J* 329 (2004): 883.

15. Brink, S. "Unlocking the Heart's Secrets." *U.S. News and World Report* 125 (1998): 56–99.

16. Kannel, W.B. "Clinical Misconceptions Dispelled by Epidemiological Research." *Circulation* 92 (1995): 3350–3360.

17. Kannel, W.B., T.R. Dawber, A. Kagan, et al. "Factors of Risk in the Development of Coronary Heart Disease—Six-year Follow-up Experience. The Framingham Study." *Ann Intern Med* 55 (1961): 33–50.

18. Mehta, N.J., and I.A. Khan. "Cardiology's 10 Greatest Discoveries of the 20th Century." *Tex Heart Inst J* 29:3 (2002): 164–171.

19. Hickey, S., and H. Roberts. *Ascorbate: The Science of Vitamin C.* Lulu Press, 2004.

20. Vinten-Johansen, P., et al. *Cholera, Chloroform, and the Science of Medicine: A Life of John Snow.* New York, NY: Oxford University Press, 2003.

21. Brody, H., M.R. Rip, P. Vinten-Johansen, et al. "Map-making and Myth-making in Broad Street: The London Cholera Epidemic, 1854." *Lancet* 356:9 223 (2000): 64–68.

22. The Committee on Scientific Inquiries of the General Board of Health, Metropolitan Commission of Sewers (1854).

23. Seaman, V. "An Inquiry into the Cause of the Prevalence of Yellow Fever in New York." *The Medical Repository, New York* 1 (1798): 315–372.

24. Stevenson, L.G. "Putting Disease on the Map: The Early Use of Spot Maps in Yellow Fever." *J Hist Med* 20 (1965): 227–261.

25. Halliday, S. *The Great Stink of London: Sir Joseph Bazalgette and the Cleansing of the Victorian Metropolis.* Stroud, England: Sutton, 2001.

26. Hickey, S., and H. Roberts. *Cancer: Nutrition and Survival.* Lulu Press, 2005. Hickey, S., H. Roberts, R.F. Cathcart. "Dynamic Flow." *J Orthomolecular Med* 20:4 (2005): 237–244.

27. Le Fanu, J. *Rise and Fall of Modern Medicine.* London, England: Little Brown, 1999.

28. Feynman, R. (1974) "Cargo Cult Science." (Cal Tech Commencement Address.) In Feynman, R., and R. Leyton. *Surely You're Joking, Mr Feynman!* New York, NY: W.W. Norton, 1997.

29. Spiro, H. "Peptic Ulcer is Not a Disease, Only a Sign! Stress is a Factor in More Than a Few Dyspeptics." *Psychosom Med* 62:2 (2000): 186–187. Sapolsky, R.M. *Why Zebras Don't Get Ulcers,* 3rd ed. New York, NY: Owl Books, 2004.

30. Caldwell, M.T., R.C. Stuart, P.J. Byrne, et al. "Microvascular Changes in Experimental Gastric Stress Ulceration: The Influence of Allopurinol, Cimetidine, and Misoprostol." *J Surg Res* 55:2 (1993): 135–139. Yi, I., M.E. Bays, F.K. Stephan. "Stress Ulcers in Rats: The Role of Food Intake, Body Weight, and Time of Day." *Physiol Behav* 54:2 (1993): 375–381. Porter, W., et al. "Some Experimental Observations on the Gastrointestinal Lesions in Behaviourally Conditioned Monkeys." *Psychosom Med* 20 (1958): 379.

31. Guyton, A.C. *Textbook of Medical Physiology.* Philadelphia, PA: W.B. Saunders, 1971.

32. Ford, A.C., B.C. Delaney, D. Forman, et al. "Eradication Therapy for Peptic Ulcer Disease in *Helicobacter pylori* Positive Patients." *Cochrane Database Syst Rev* 2 (April 2006): CD003840.

33. Robillard, N. *Heartburn Cured: The Low-Carb Miracle.* Watertown, MA: Self Health Publishing, 2005.

34. Popper, K. *Logic of Scientific Discovery.* London, England: Routledge Classics, 1959. Popper, K. *Conjectures and Refutations: The Growth of Scientific Knowledge.* London, England: Routledge, 1963.

35. Gigerenzer, G. *Reckoning with Risk.* New York, NY: Penguin, 2003.

36. Douglas, R.M., H. Hemilä, E. Chalker, et al. "Vitamin C for Preventing and Treating the Common Cold." (Review.) *Cochrane Library Issue* 3 (2007).

37. Schwartz, A.R., Y. Togo, R.B. Hornick, et al. "Evaluation of the Efficacy of Ascorbic Acid in Prophylaxis of Induced Rhinovirus 44 Infection in Man." *J Infect Dis* 128 (1973): 500–505. Walker, G., M.L. Bynoe, D.A. Tyrrell. "Trial of Ascorbic Acid in Prevention of Colds." *Br Med J* 1 (1967): 603–606. Karlowski, T.R., T.C. Chalmers, L.D. Frenkel, et al. "Ascorbic Acid for the Common Cold." *JAMA* 231 (1975): 1038–1042.

38. Higgins, R. "Doses Too Small." In Douglas, R.M., H. Hemilä, E. Chalker, et al. "Vitamin C for Preventing and Treating the Common Cold." (Review.) *Cochrane Library Issue* 3 (2007).

39. Cathcart, R.F. "The Three Faces of Vitamin C." *J Orthomolecular Med* 7:4 (1993): 197–200.

40. Cathcart, R.F. "Vitamin C: The Non-toxic, Non-rate-limited, Antioxidant Free Radical Scavenger." *Med Hypotheses* 18 (1985): 61–77.

41. Cathcart, R.F. "Vitamin C, Titrating to Bowel Tolerance, Anascorbemia, and Acute Induced Scurvy." *Med Hypotheses* 7 (1981): 1359–1376. Available online at: http://www.doctoryourself.com/titration.html.

42. Anderson, T.W., G. Suranyi, G.H. Beaton. "The Effect on Winter Illness of Large Doses of Vitamin C." *Can Med Assoc J* 111 (1974): 31–36.

43. Hickey, S., and H. Roberts. *Ascorbate: The Science of Vitamin C.* Lulu Press, 2004.

44. Angell, M. *The Truth About the Drug Companies.* New York, NY: Random House, 2004. Goozner, M. *The $800 Million Pill.* Berkeley, CA: University of California Press, 2004.

45. Sardi, Bill. Personal communication (2006).

46. Taylor, H. "Reputation of Pharmaceutical Companies, While Still Poor, Improves for Second Year in a Row." *Healthcare News* 6:5 (May 2006). Harris Interactive. http://www.harrisinteractive.com.

47. Weber, L.J. *Profits Before People? Ethical Standards and the Marketing of Prescription Drugs.* Bloomington, IN: Indiana University Press, 2006. Henry J. Kaiser Family Foundation. "Views on Prescription Drugs and the Pharmaceutical Industry." *Kaiser Health Report* (January/February 2005). Available online at: www.kff.org.

48. Kalokerinos, A. *Every Second Child.* Chicago, IL: Keats Publishing, 1991.

49. Everson, T.C., and W.H. Cole. *Spontaneous Regression of Cancer.* Philadelphia, PA: W.B. Saunders, 1966. Boyd, W. *Spontaneous Regression of Cancer.* Springfield, IL: Charles C. Thomas, 1966.

50. Kienle, G.S., and H. Kiene. "The Powerful Placebo Effect: Fact or Fiction?" *J Clin Epidemiol* 50:12 (1997): 1311–1318.

51. Levine, M.E., R.M. Stern, K.L. Koch. "The Effects of Manipulating Expectations through Placebo and Nocebo Administration on Gastric Tachyarrhythmia and Motion-induced Nausea." *Psychosom Med* 68 (2006): 478–486.

52. Hróbjartsson, A., and P.C. Gotzsche. "Is the Placebo Powerless? An Analysis of Clinical Trials Comparing Placebo with No Treatment." *N Engl J Med* 344:21 (2001): 1594–1602. [Erratum: *N Engl J Med* 345:4 (2001): 304.]

53. Spiegel, D., H. Kraemer, R.W. Carlson. "Is the Placebo Powerless?" *N Engl J Med* 345:17 (2001): 1276. Klosterhalfen, S., and P. Enck. "Psychobiology of the Placebo Response." *Auton Neurosci* 125:1–2 (2006): 94–99.

54. Kolata, G. "Placebo Effect is More Myth Than Science, a Study Says." *The New York Times* (May 24, 2001).

55. Cameron, E., and L. Pauling. *Cancer and Vitamin C.* Philadelphia, PA: Camino Books, 1993. Cameron, E., and L. Pauling. "Supplemental Ascorbate in the Supportive Treatment of Cancer: Reevaluation of Prolongation of Survival Times in Terminal Human Cancer." *Proc Natl Acad Sci USA* 75 (1978):

4538–4542. Hoffer, A. *Vitamin C and Cancer: Discovery, Recovery, Controversy.* Kingston, ON, Canada: Quarry Press, 2000. Murata, A., F. Morishige, H. Yamaguchi. "Prolongation of Survival Times of Terminal Cancer Patients by Administration of Large Doses of Ascorbate." *Intl J Vitamin Nutr Res Suppl* 23 (1982): 101–113.

56. Matre, D., K.L. Casey, S. Knardahl. "Placebo-induced Changes in Spinal Cord Pain Processing." *J Neurosci* 26:2 (2006): 559–563. Dworkin, R.H., J. Katz, M.J. Gitlin. "Placebo Response in Clinical Trials of Depression and Its Implications for Research on Chronic Neuropathic Pain." *Neurology* 65:12 Suppl 4 (2005): S7–S19.

57. Benedetti, F., H.S. Mayberg, T.D. Wager, et al. "Neurobiological Mechanisms of the Placebo Effect." *J Neurosci* 25:45 (2005): 10390–10402.

58. Ellis, S.J., and R.F. Adams. "The Cult of the Double-blind Placebo-controlled Trial." *Br J Clin Pract* 51:1 (1997): 36–39.

59. Williams, R.J. *Biochemical Individuality: The Basis for the Genetotrophic Concept.* New Canaan, CT: Keats, 1998.

60. Sech, S.M., J.D. Montoya, P.A. Bernier, et al. "The So-called 'Placebo Effect' in Benign Prostatic Hyperplasia Treatment Trials Represents Partially a Conditional Regression to the Mean Induced by Censoring." *Urology* 51:2 (1998): 242–250.

61. Galton, F. "Regression Towards Mediocrity in Hereditary Stature." *J Anthropol Inst* 15 (1886): 246–263.

62. Morton, V., and D.J. Torgerson. "Effect of Regression to the Mean on Decision Making in Health Care." *Br Med J* 326:7398 (2003): 1083–1084.

63. Tversky, A., and D. Kahneman. "Judgement Under Uncertainty: Heuristics and Biases." *Science* 185 (1974): 1124–1131.

64. Bellia, V., S. Battaglia, F. Catalano, et al. "Aging and Disability Affect Misdiagnosis of COPD in Elderly Asthmatics: The SARA Study." *Chest* 123:4 (2003): 1066–1072. Baxter, A.J., and C.S. Gray. "Diastolic Heart Failure in Older People—Myth or Lost Tribe?" *Clin Med* 2:6 (2002): 539–543. Porta, M., S. Costafreda, N. Malats, et al. "Validity of the Hospital Discharge Diagnosis in Epidemiologic Studies of Biliopancreatic Pathology. PANKRAS II Study Group." *Eur J Epidemiol* 16:6 (2000): 533–541.

65. Duda, S., C. Aliferis, R. Miller, et al. "Extracting Drug-Drug Interaction Articles from MEDLINE to Improve the Content of Drug Databases." *AMIA Annu Symp Proc* (2005): 216–220. Barbanoj, M.J., R.M. Antonijoan, J. Riba, et al. "Quantifying Drug-Drug Interactions in Pharmaco-EEG." *Clin EEG Neurosci* 37:2 (2006): 108–120.

66. Gøtzsche, P.C. "Believability of Relative Risks and Odds Ratios in Abstracts: Cross-sectional Study." *Br Med J* 333 (2006): 231–234.

67. Scherer, R.W., P. Langenberg, E. von Elm. "Full Publication of Results Initially Presented in Abstracts." *Cochrane Database Methodol Rev* 2 (2005): MR000005.

68. Gøtzsche, P.C. "Methodology and Overt and Hidden Bias in Reports of 196 Double-blind Trials of Nonsteroidal, Anti-inflammatory Drugs in Rheumatoid Arthritis." *Controlled Clin Trials* 10 (1989): 31–56. [Amended: *Controlled Clin Trials* 10 (1989): 356.]

69. Chan, A.W., A. Hróbjartsson, B. Tendal, et al. "Pre-specifying sample size calculations and statistical analyses in randomised trials: Comparison of protocols to publications." XIII Cochrane Colloquium, Melbourne, Australia, October 22-26, 2005, p. 66.

70 Chan, A.W., A. Hróbjartsson, M.T. Haahr, et al. "Empirical Evidence for Selective Reporting of Outcomes in Randomized Trials: Comparison of Protocols to Published Articles." *JAMA* 291 (2004): 2457–2465.

71. Chan, A.W., K. Krleza-Jeric, I. Schmid, et al. "Outcome Reporting Bias in Randomized Trials Funded by the Canadian Institutes of Health Research." *Can Med Assoc J* 171 (2004): 735–740.

72. Chan, A.W., and D.G. Altman. "Identifying Outcome Reporting Bias in Randomised Trials on PubMed: Review of Publications and Survey of Authors." *Br Med J* 330 (2005): 753. "Reporting of Trial Outcomes is Incomplete and Biased." (Editorial.) *Br Med J* 330 (2005).

73. Bjelakovic, G., D. Nikolova, L.L. Gluud, et al. "Mortality in Randomized Trials of Antioxidant Supplements for Primary and Secondary Prevention: Systematic Review and Meta-analysis." *JAMA* 297 (2007): 842–857.

74. Hickey, S., L. Noriega, H. Roberts. "Poor Methodology in Meta-analysis of Vitamins." *J Orthomolecular Med* 22:1 (2007): 8–10.

Chapter 5: The Need for Antioxidants

1. Halliwell, B., and J.M.C. Gutteridge. *Free Radicals in Biology and Medicine.* Oxford, England: Oxford University Press, 1999.

2. Packer, L., and C. Colman. *The Antioxidant Miracle.* New York, NY: Wiley, 1999.

3. Linster, C.L., T.A. Gomez, K.C. Christensen, et al. "Arabidopsis VTC2 Encodes a GDP-L-galactose Phosphorylase, the Last Unknown Enzyme in the Smirnoff-Wheeler Pathway to Ascorbic Acid in Plants." *J Biol Chem* 282:26 (2007): 18879–18885.

4. Bors, W., and G.R. Buettner. "The Vitamin C Radical and Its Reactions." In Packer, L., and J. Fuchs (eds.). *Vitamin C in Health and Disease.* New York, NY: Marcel Dekker, 1997, pp. 75–94.

5. Kubin, A., K. Kaudela, R. Jindra, et al. "Dehydroascorbic Acid in Urine as a Possible Indicator of Surgical Stress." *Ann Nutr Metab* 47:1 (2003): 1–5.

6. Sinclair, A.J., P.B. Taylor. J. Lunec, et al. "Low Plasma Ascorbate Levels in Patients with Type 2 Diabetes Mellitus Consuming Adequate Dietary Vitamin C." *Diabet Med* 11:9 (1994): 893–898.

7. Rusakow, L.S., J. Han, M.A. Hayward, et al. "Pulmonary Oxygen Toxicity in Mice is Characterized by Alterations in Ascorbate Redox Status." *J Appl Physiol* 79:5 (1995): 1769–1776.

8. Obrosova, I.G., L. Fathallah, E. Liu, et al. "Early Oxidative Stress in the Diabetic Kidney: Effect of DL-Alpha-lipoic Acid." *Free Radic Biol Med* 34:2 (2003): 186–195. Jiang, Q., J. Lykkesfeldt, M.K. Shigenaga, et al. "Gamma-tocopherol Supplementation Inhibits Protein Nitration and Ascorbate Oxidation in Rats with Inflammation." *Free Radic Biol Med* 33:11 (2002): 1534–1542. Simoes, S.I., C.V. Eleuterio, M.E. Cruz, et al. "Biochemical Changes in Arthritic Rats: Dehydroascorbic and Ascorbic Acid Levels." *Eur J Pharm Sci* 18:2 (2003): 185–189.

9. Schafer, F., and G.R. Buettner. "Redox Environment of the Cell as Viewed Through the Redox State of the Glutathione Disulfide/Glutathione Couple." *Free Radic Biol Med* 30:11 (2001): 1191–1202.

10. Montecinos, V., P. Guzmán, V. Barra, et al. (2007) "Vitamin C is an Essential Antioxidant that Enhances Survival of Oxidatively Stressed Human Vascular Endothelial Cells in the Presence of a Vast Molar Excess of Glutathione." *J Biol Chem* 282:21 (May 2007): 15506–15515.

11. Cathcart, R.F. "Vitamin C: The Nontoxic, Non-rate-limited, Antioxidant Free Radical Scavenger." *Med Hypotheses* 18 (1985): 61–77.

12. Hickey, S., R.F. Cathcart, H.J. Roberts. "Dynamic Flow." *J Orthomolecular Med* 20:4 (2005): 237–244.

13. Vitamin C Foundation. http://www.vitamincfoundation.org/surefire.htm. Accessed April 7, 2007.

14. Chakrabarti, B., and S. Banerjee. "Dehydroascorbic Acid Level in Blood of Patients Suffering from Various Infectious Diseases." *Proc Soc Exp Biol Med* 88 (1955): 581–583.

15. May, J.M., Z. Qu, X. Li. "Requirement for GSH in Recycling of Ascorbic Acid in Endothelial Cells." *Biochem Pharmacol* 62:7 (2001): 873–881.

Vethanayagam, J.G., E.H. Green, R.C. Rose, et al. "Glutathione-dependent Ascorbate Recycling Activity of Rat Serum Albumin." *Free Radic Biol Med* 26 (1999): 1591–1598. Mendiratta, S., Z.C. Qu, J.M. May. "Enzyme-dependent Ascorbate Recycling in Human Erythrocytes: Role of Thioredoxin Reductase." *Free Radic Biol Med* 25 (1998): 221–228.

16. Jacob, R.A. "The Integrated Antioxidant System." *Nutr Res* 15 (1995): 755–766. Lewin, S. *Vitamin C: Its Molecular Biology and Medical Potential.* New York, NY: Academic Press, 1976. Cathcart, R.F. "A Unique Function for Ascorbate." *Med Hypotheses* 35 (1991): 32–37. Pauling, L. *General Chemistry.* New York, NY: Dover, 1988.

Chapter 6: Infectious Diseases

1. Bhopal, R.S. "Generating Health from Patterns of Disease." *Proc R Coll Physicians Edinburgh* 31 (2001): 293–298.

2. Falco, V., F. de Silva, J. Alegre, et al. "*Legionella pneumophila:* A Cause of Severe Community-acquired Pneumonia." *Chest* 100 (1991): 1007–1011. el-Ebiary, M., X. Sarmiento, A. Torres, et al. "Prognostic Factors of Severe *Legionella* Pneumonia Requiring Admission to ICU." *Am J Respir Crit Care Med* 156 (1997): 1467–1472. Marston, B.J., H.B. Lipman, R.F. Breiman. "Surveillance for Legionnaires' Disease: Risk Factors for Morbidity and Mortality." *Arch Intern Med* 154 (1994): 2417–2422.

3. England, A.C., D.W. Fraser, B.D. Plikaytis, et al. "Sporadic Legionellosis in the United States: The First Thousand Cases." *Ann Intern Med* 94 (1981): 164–170. Lettinga, K.D., A. Verbon, G.J. Weverling, et al. "Legionnaires' Disease at a Dutch Flower Show: Prognostic Factors and Impact of Therapy." *Emerg Infect Dis* 8:12 (December 2002): 1448–1454.

4. Levy, T.E. *Vitamin C, Infectious Disease and Toxins.* Xlibris, 2002.

5. U.S. Department of Health and Human Services. *Vital Statistics of the U.S.,* Vol. 2. Washington, DC: U.S. Department of Health and Human Services, 1989.

6. Cathcart, R.F. "Vitamin C Function in AIDS." *Medical Tribune* (July 13, 1983). Cathcart, R.F. "Vitamin C in the Treatment of Acquired Immune Deficiency Syndrome (AIDS)." *Med Hypotheses* 14 (1984): 423–433.

7. Brighthope, I., and P. Fitzgerald. *The AIDS Fighters.* New Canaan, CT: Keats, 1987.

8. Hickey, S., and H. Roberts. *Ascorbate: The Science of Vitamin C.* Lulu Press, 2004.

9. Sardi, B. "Global Battle Erupts Over Vitamin Supplements." www.lewrockwell.com. May 16, 2005.

10. Fuller, J.G. *Fever! The Hunt for a New Killer Virus.* Pleasantville, NY: Reader's Digest Press, 1974.

11. Klenner, F. "The Significance of High Daily Intake of Ascorbic Acid in Preventive Medicine." In Williams, R., and D.K. Kalita (eds.). *Physician's Handbook on Orthomolecular Medicine,* 3rd ed. New York, NY: Pergamon, 1977.

12. Cathcart, R.F. "Clinical Trial of Vitamin C." (Letter to the Editor.) *Medical Tribune* (June 25, 1975).

13. Cathcart, R.F. "Vitamin C Titrating to Bowel Tolerance, Anascorbemia and Acute Induced Scurvy." *Med Hypotheses* 7 (1981): 1359–1376.

14. Levy, T.E. *Vitamin C, Infectious Disease and Toxins.* Xlibris, 2002. Hoffer, A., and M. Walker. *Putting It All Together: The New Orthomolecular Nutrition.* New Canaan, CT: Keats, 1978.

15. Cathcart, R.F. Unpublished paper on AIDS. (Letter to Editor.) Critical Path Project, 1992.

16. Kalokerinos, A. *Every Second Child.* Melbourne, Australia: Thomas Nelson, 1974.

Chapter 7: Cancer and Vitamin C

1. Nakagaki, T., H. Yamada, A. Tóth. "Intelligence: Maze-solving by an Amoeboid Organism." *Nature* 407 (2000): 470.

2. Shaffer, B.M. "Secretion of Cyclic AMP Induced by Cyclic AMP in the Cellular Slime Mould *Dictyostelium discoideum.*" *Nature* 255 (1975): 549–552.

3. Hardman, A.M., G.S. Stewart, P. Williams. "Quorum Sensing and the Cell-Cell Communication Dependent Regulation of Gene Expression in Pathogenic and Non-pathogenic Bacteria." *Antonie Van Leeuwenhoek J Microbiol Serol* 74 (1998): 199–210. Fuqua, C., and E.P. Greenberg. "Self Perception in Bacteria: Quorum Sensing with Acylated Homoserine Lactones." *Curr Opin Microbiol* 1 (1998): 183–189.

4. Lewis, K. "Programmed Death in Bacteria." *Microbiol Molec Biol Rev* 64:3 (2000): 503–514.

5. Everson, T.C., and W.H. Cole. *Spontaneous Regression of Cancer.* Philadelphia, PA: W.B. Saunders, 1966. Boyd, W. *Spontaneous Regression of Cancer.* Springfield, IL: Charles C. Thomas, 1966.

6. Voght, A. "On the Vitamin C Treatment of Chronic Leukemias." *Deutsche Med Wochenschr* 14 (April 1940): 369–372.

7. McCormick, W.J. "Cancer: The Preconditioning Factor in Pathogenesis."

Arch Pediatr 71 (1954): 313–322. McCormick, W.J. "Cancer: A Collagen Disease, Secondary to a Nutritional Deficiency?" *Arch Pediatr* 76 (1959): 166–171.

8. Stone, I. *The Healing Factor: "Vitamin C" Against Disease.* New York, NY: Grosset and Dunlap, 1972.

9. Greer, E. "Alcoholic Cirrhosis: Complicated by Polycythemia Vera and Then Myelogenous Leukemia and Tolerance of Large Doses of Vitamin C." *Medical Times* 82 (1954): 765–768.

10. Cameron, E., and D. Rotman. "Ascorbic Acid, Cell Proliferation, and Cancer." *Lancet* 1 (1972): 542. Cameron, E., and L. Pauling. "Ascorbic Acid and the Glycosaminoglycans: An Orthomolecular Approach to Cancer and Other Diseases." *Oncology* 27 (1973): 181–192. Cameron, E., and A. Campbell. "The Orthomolecular Treatment of Cancer II. Clinical Trial of High-dose Ascorbic Acid Supplements in Advanced Human Cancer." *Chem Biol Interact* 9 (1974): 285–315. Cameron, E., and L. Pauling. "Supplemental Ascorbate in the Supportive Treatment of Cancer: Prolongation of Survival Times in Terminal Human Cancer." *Proc Natl Acad Sci USA* 73 (1976): 3685–3689. Cameron, E., and L. Pauling. "Supplemental Ascorbate in the Supportive Treatment of Cancer: Reevaluation of Prolongation of Survival Times in Terminal Human Cancer." *Proc Natl Acad Sci USA* 75 (1978): 4538–4542. Cameron, E. "Vitamin C for Cancer." *N Engl J Med* 302 (1980): 299. Cameron, E., and A. Campbell. "Innovation vs. Quality Control: An 'Unpublishable' Clinical Trial of Supplemental Ascorbate in Incurable Cancer." *Med Hypotheses* 36 (1991): 185–189.

11. Campbell, A., T. Jack, E. Cameron. "Reticulum Cell Sarcoma: Two Complete 'Spontaneous' Regressions in Response to High-dose Ascorbic Acid Therapy. A Report on Subsequent Progress." *Oncology* 48 (1991): 495–497.

12. Pauling, L. Personal communication.

13. Hickey, S., and H. Roberts. "Selfish Cells: Cancer as Microevolution." *J Orthomolecular Med* (2007) (in press).

14. Hickey, S., and H. Roberts. *Cancer: Nutrition and Survival.* Lulu Press, 2005.

15. Schafer, F.Q., and G.R. Buettner. "Redox Environment of the Cell as Viewed through the Redox State of the Glutathione Disulfide/Glutathione Couple." *Free Radic Biol Med* 30:11 (2001): 1191–1212.

16. Matheu, A., A. Maraver, P. Klatt, et al. "Delayed Ageing through Damage Protection by the *Arf/p53* Pathway." *Nature* 448:7151 (2007): 375–381.

17. Hickey, S., and H. Roberts. *Ascorbate: The Science of Vitamin C.* Lulu Press, 2004.

18. Gunn, H. "The Use of Antioxidants with Chemotherapy and Radiotherapy in Cancer Treatment: A Review." *J Orthomolecular Med* 19:4 (2004): 246. Stoute, J.A. "The Use of Vitamin C with Chemotherapy in Cancer Treatment: An Annotated Bibliography." *J Orthomolecular Med* 19:4 (2004): 198. Hoffer, A. "The Use of Vitamin C and Other Antioxidants with Chemotherapy and Radiotherapy in Cancer Treatment." *J Orthomolecular Med* 19:4 (2004): 195.

19. Hickey, S., and H. Roberts. *The Cancer Breakthrough*. Lulu Press, 2007.

Chapter 8: Heart Disease

1. Hoffer, A., and M. Walker. *Putting It All Together: The New Orthomolecular Nutrition*. New Canaan, CT: Keats, 1978.

2. Yavorsky, M., P. Almaden, C.G. King. "The Vitamin C Content of Human Tissues." *J Biol Chem* 106:2 (1934): 525–529.

3. Lewin, S. *Vitamin C: Its Molecular Biology and Medicinal Potential*. New York, NY: Academic Press, 1976.

4. McCormick, W.J. "Coronary Thrombosis: A New Concept of Mechanism and Etiology." *Clin Med* 4:7 (July 1957). Paterson, J.C. "Some Factors in the Causation of Intimal Hemorrhages and in the Precipitation of Coronary Thrombi." *Can Med Assoc J* (February 1941): 114–120. Paterson, J.C. "Capillary Rupture with Intimal Haemorrhage in the Causation of Cerebral Vascular Lesions." *Arch Pathol* 29 (1940): 345–354. Willis, G.C. "An Experimental Study of the Intimal Ground Substance in Atherosclerosis." *Can Med Assoc J* 69 (1953): 17–22. Willis, G.C. "The Reversibility of Atherosclerosis." *Can Med Assoc J* 77 (1957): 106–109. Willis, G.C., A.W. Light, W.S. Cow. "Serial Arteriography in Atherosclerosis." *Can Med Assoc J* 71 (1954): 562–568. Willis, G.C., and S. Fishman. "Ascorbic Acid Content of Human Arterial Tissue." *Can Med Assoc J* 72 (April 1955): 500–503.

5. Rath, M., and L. Pauling. "Immunological Evidence for the Accumulation of Lipoprotein(a) in the Atherosclerotic Lesion of the Hypoascorbemic Guinea Pig." *Proc Natl Acad Sci* 87:23 (December 1990): 9388–9390. Rath, M., and L. Pauling. "Solution to the Puzzle of Human Cardiovascular Disease: Its Primary Cause is Ascorbate Deficiency, Leading to the Deposition of Lipoprotein(a) and Fibrinogen/Fibrin in the Vascular Wall." *J Orthomolecular Med* 6 (1991): 125–134. Pauling, L., and M. Rath. "Prevention and Treatment of Occlusive Cardiovascular Disease with Ascorbate and Substances that Inhibit the Binding of Lipoprotein(A)." U.S. Patent 5,278,189 (1994). Pauling, L., and M. Rath. "Use of Ascorbate and Tranexamic Acid Solution for Organ and Blood Vessel Treatment Prior to Transplantation." U.S. Patent 5,230,996 (1993). Rath, M., and A. Niedzwiecki. "Nutritional Supplement Program Halts

Progression of Early Coronary Atherosclerosis Documented by Ultrafast Computed Tomography." *J Appl Nutr* 48 (1996): 68–78.

6. Hickey, S., and H. Roberts. *Ascorbate: The Science of Vitamin C.* Lulu Press, 2004.

7. Harjai, K.J. "Potential New Cardiovascular Risk Factors: Left Ventricular Hypertrophy, Homocysteine, Lipoprotein(a), Triglycerides, Oxidative Stress, and Fibrinogen." *Ann Intern Med* 131 (1999): 376–386. Grant, P.J. "The Genetics of Atherothrombotic Disorders: A Clinician's View." *J Thromb Haemost* 1 (2003): 1381–1390. Maas, R., and R.H. Boger. "Old and New Cardiovascular Risk Factors: From Unresolved Issues to New Opportunities." *Atheroscler Suppl* 4 (2003): 5–17. Dominiczak, M.H. "Risk Factors for Coronary Disease: The Time for a Paradigm Shift?" *Clin Chem Lab Med* 39 (2001): 907–919. Frostegard, J. "Autoimmunity, Oxidized LDL and Cardiovascular Disease." *Autoimmun Rev* 1 (2002): 233–237.

8. Harrison, D.G., H. Cai, U. Landmesser, et al. "Interactions of Angiotensin II with NAD(P)H Oxidase, Oxidant Stress and Cardiovascular Disease." *J Renin Angiotensin Aldosterone Syst* 4 (2003): 51–61. Cuff, C.A., D. Kothapalli, E. Azonobi, et al. "The Adhesion Receptor CD44 Promotes Atherosclerosis by Mediating Inflammatory Cell Recruitment and Vascular Cell Activation." *J Clin Invest* 108 (2001): 1031–1040. Huang, Y., L. Song, S. Wu, et al. "Oxidized LDL Differentially Regulates MMP-1 and TIMP-1 Expression in Vascular Endothelial Cells." *Atherosclerosis* 156 (2001): 119–125. McIntyre, T.M., S.M. Prescott, A.S. Weyrich, et al. "Cell-Cell Interactions: Leukocyte-Endothelial Interactions." *Curr Opin Hematol* 10 (2003): 150–158.

9. Gonzalez, M.A., and A.P. Selwyn. "Endothelial Function, Inflammation, and Prognosis in Cardiovascular Disease." *Am J Med* 115 (2003): 99S–106S.

10. Weber, C., E. Wolfgang, K. Weber, et al. "Increased Adhesiveness of Isolated Monocytes to Epithelium is Prevented by Vitamin C Intake in Smokers." *Circulation* 93 (1996): 1488–1492.

11. Scribner, A.W., J. Loscalzo, C. Napoli. "The Effect of Angiotensin-converting Enzyme Inhibition on Endothelial Function and Oxidant Stress." *Eur J Pharmacol* 482 (2003): 95–99. Elisaf, M. "Effects of Fibrates on Serum Metabolic Parameters." *Curr Med Res Opin* 18 (2002): 269–276. Vane, J.R., and R.M. Botting. "The Mechanism of Action of Aspirin." *Thromb Res* 110 (2003): 255–258. Carneado, J., M. Alvarez de Sotomayor, C. Perez-Guerrero, et al. "Simvastatin Improves Endothelial Function in Spontaneously Hypertensive Rats through a Superoxide Dismutase Mediated Antioxidant Effect." *J Hypertens* 20 (2002): 429–437. Erkkila, L., M. Jauhiainen, K. Laitinen, et al. "Effect of Simvastatin, an Established Lipid-lowering Drug, on Pulmonary *Chlamydia*

pneumoniae Infection in Mice." *Antimicrob Agents Chemother* 49:9 (2005): 3959–3962.

12. Stone, I. *The Healing Factor: Vitamin C Against Disease.* New York, NY: Putnam, 1974. Hickey, S., and H. Roberts. *Ascorbate: The Science of Vitamin C.* Lulu Press, 2004. Levy, T.E. *Stop America's #1 Killer.* LivOn Books, 2006.

13. Salzar, R.S., M.J. Thubrikar, R.T. Eppink. "Pressure-induced Mechanical Stress in the Carotid Artery Bifurcation: A Possible Correlation to Atherosclerosis." *J Biomech* 28:11 (1995): 1333–1340.

14. D'Orleans-Juste, P., J. Labonte, G. Bkaily, et al. "Function of the Endothelin(B) Receptor in Cardiovascular Physiology and Pathophysiology." *Pharmacol Ther* 95 (2002): 221–238. Annuk, M., M. Zilmer, B. Fellstrom. "Endothelium-dependent Vasodilation and Oxidative Stress in Chronic Renal Failure: Impact on Cardiovascular Disease." *Kidney Intl Suppl* 84 (2003): S50–S53. Egashira, K. "Clinical Importance of Endothelial Function in Arteriosclerosis and Ischemic Heart Disease." *Circ J* 66 (2002): 529–533. Luscher, T.F., F.C. Tanner, M.R. Tschudi, et al. "Endothelial Dysfunction in Coronary Artery Disease." *Annu Rev Med* 44 (1993): 395–418.

15. Gong, L., G.M. Pitari, S. Schulz, et al. "Nitric Oxide Signaling: Systems Integration of Oxygen Balance in Defense of Cell Integrity." *Curr Opin Hematol* 11 (2004): 7–14. Sumpio, B.E., J.T. Riley, A. Dardik. "Cells in Focus: Endothelial Cell." *Intl J Biochem Cell Biol* 34 (2002): 1508–1512. Ando, J., and A. Kamiya. "Blood Flow and Vascular Endothelial Cell Function." *Front Med Biol Eng* 5 (1993): 245–264.

16. Higgins, J.P. "Can Angiotensin-converting Enzyme Inhibitors Reverse Atherosclerosis?" *South Med J* 96 (2003): 569–579. Harrison, D.G., and H. Cai. "Endothelial Control of Vasomotion and Nitric Oxide Production." *Cardiol Clin* 21 (2003): 289–302. Stankevicius, E., E. Kevelaitis, E. Vainorius, et al. "Role of Nitric Oxide and Other Endothelium-derived Factors." *Medicina (Kaunas)* 39 (2003): 333–341. Vane, J.R., and R.M. Botting. "Secretory Functions of the Vascular Endothelium." *J Physiol Pharmacol* 43 (1992): 195–207. Chauhan, S.D., H. Nilsson, A. Ahluwalia, et al. "Release of C-type Natriuretic Peptide Accounts for the Biological Activity of Endothelium-derived Hyperpolarizing Factor." *Proc Natl Acad Sci USA* 100 (2003): 1426–1431.

17. Pearson, J.D. "Endothelial Cell Function and Thrombosis." *Baillieres Best Pract Res Clin Haematol* 12 (1999): 329–341. Huber, D., E.M. Cramer, J.E. Kaufmann, et al. "Tissue-type Plasminogen Activator (t-PA) is Stored in Weibel-Palade Bodies in Human Endothelial Cells Both in Vitro and in Vivo." *Blood* 99 (2002): 3637–3645.

18. Vallance, P., J. Collier, S. Moncada. "Effects of Endothelium-derived Nitric Oxide on Peripheral Arteriolar Tone in Man." *Lancet* 2 (1989): 997–1000.

19. Major, T.C., R.W. Overhiser, R.L. Panek. "Evidence for NO Involvement in Regulating Vascular Reactivity in Balloon-injured Rat Carotid Artery." *Am J Physiol* 269 (1995): H988–H996.

20. Taddei, S., A. Virdis, L. Ghiadoni, et al. "Vitamin C Improves Endothelium-dependent Vasodilation by Restoring Nitric Oxide Activity in Essential Hypertension." *Circulation* 97:22 (1998): 2222–2229.

21. Hampl, V. "Nitric Oxide and Regulation of Pulmonary Vessels." *Cesk Fysiol* 49 (2000): 22–29.

22. Stankevicius, E., E. Kevelaitis, E. Vainorius, et al. "Role of Nitric Oxide and Other Endothelium-derived Factors." *Medicina* (*Kaunas*) 39 (2003): 333–341.

23. De Nigris, F., L.O. Lerman, W.S. Ignarro, et al. "Beneficial Effects of Antioxidants and L-Arginine on Oxidation-sensitive Gene Expression and Endothelial NO Synthase Activity at Sites of Disturbed Shear Stress." *Proc Natl Acad Sci USA* 100:3 (February 2003): 1420–1425.

24. Shmit, E. "Antioxidant Vitamins May Prevent Blood Vessel Blockage and Protect Against Cardiovascular Disease." *UCLA News* (January 15, 2003).

25. Watanabe, T., R. Pakala, T. Katagiri, et al. "Monocyte Chemotactic Protein 1 Amplifies Serotonin-induced Vascular Smooth Muscle Cell Proliferation." *J Vasc Res* 38 (2001): 341–349. Rainger, G.E., and G.B. Nash. "Cellular Pathology of Atherosclerosis: Smooth Muscle Cells Prime Cocultured Endothelial Cells for Enhanced Leukocyte Adhesion." *Circ Res* 88 (2001): 615–622. Desai, A., H.A. Lankford, J.S. Warren. "Homocysteine Augments Cytokine-induced Chemokine Expression in Human Vascular Smooth Muscle Cells: Implications for Atherogenesis." *Inflammation* 25 (2001): 179–186.

26. Libby, P. "Changing Concepts of Atherogenesis." *J Intern Med* 247 (2000): 349–358.

27. Kockx, M.M., and A.G. Herman. "Apoptosis in Atherosclerosis: Beneficial or Detrimental?" *Cardiovasc Res* 45 (2000): 736–746. Gronholdt, M.L., S. Dalager-Pedersen, E. Falk. "Coronary Atherosclerosis: Determinants of Plaque Rupture." *Eur Heart J* 19 (1998): C24–C29.

28. Bennett, M.R. "Breaking the Plaque: Evidence for Plaque Rupture in Animal Models of Atherosclerosis." *Arterioscler Thromb Vasc Biol* 22 (2002): 713–714. Bennett, M.R. "Vascular Smooth Muscle Cell Apoptosis—A Dangerous Phenomenon in Vascular Disease." *J Clin Basic Cardiol* 3 (2000): 63–65.

29. Kolodgie, F.D., H.K. Gold, A.P. Burke, et al. "Intraplaque Hemorrhage and Progression of Coronary Atheroma." *N Engl J Med* 349 (2003): 2316–2325. Fan, J., and T. Watanabe. "Inflammatory Reactions in the Pathogenesis of Atherosclerosis." *J Atheroscler Thromb* 10 (2003): 63–71.

30. Barbieri, S.S., S. Eligini, M. Brambilla, et al. "Reactive Oxygen Species Mediate Cyclooxygenase-2 Induction during Monocyte to Macrophage Differentiation: Critical Role of NADPH Oxidase." *Cardiovasc Res* 60 (2003): 187–197.

31. Carpenter, K.L., I.R. Challis, M.J. Arends. "Mildly Oxidised LDL Induces More Macrophage Death than Moderately Oxidised LDL: Roles of Peroxidation, Lipoprotein-associated Phospholipase A2 and PPARgamma." *FEBS Lett* 553 (2003): 145–150. Norata, G.D., L. Tonti, P. Roma, et al. "Apoptosis and Proliferation of Endothelial Cells in Early Atherosclerotic Lesions: Possible Role of Oxidised LDL." *Nutr Metab Cardiovasc Dis* 12 (2002): 297–305.

32. Berliner, J.A., and J.W. Heinecke. "The Role of Oxidized Lipoproteins in Atherogenesis." *Free Radical Biol Med* 20 (1996): 707–727.

33. Libby, P., and M. Aikawa. "Effects of Statins in Reducing Thrombotic Risk and Modulating Plaque Vulnerability." *Clin Cardiol* 26 (2003): I11–I14. Libby, P., and M. Aikawa. "Stabilization of Atherosclerotic Plaques: New Mechanisms and Clinical Targets." *Nat Med* 8 (2002): 1257–1262.

34. Sutter, M.C. "Lessons for Atherosclerosis Research from Tuberculosis and Peptic Ulcer." *Can Med Assoc J* 152:5 (1995): 667–670. Capron, L. "Viruses and Atherosclerosis." *Rev Prat* 40:24 (1990): 2227–2233. Benitez, R.M. "Atherosclerosis: An Infectious Disease?" *Hosp Pract (Minneapolis)* 34:9 (1999): 79–82, 85–86, 89–90. Streblow, D.N., S.L. Orloff, J.A. Nelson. "Do Pathogens Accelerate Atherosclerosis?" *J Nutr* 131:10 (2001): 2798S–2804S.

35. Mehta, J.L., T.G. Saldeen, K. Rand. "Interactive Role of Infection, Inflammation and Traditional Risk Factors in Atherosclerosis and Coronary Artery Disease." *J Am Coll Cardiol* 31:6 (1998): 1217–1225. Broxmeyer, L. "Heart Disease: The Greatest 'Risk' Factor of Them All." *Med Hypotheses* 62:5 (2004): 773–779.

36. Friedman, H.M., E.J. Macarak, R.R. MacGregor, et al. "Virus Infection of Endothelial Cells." *J Infect Dis* 143:2 (1981): 266–273. Tumilowicz, J.J., M.E. Gawlik, B.B. Powell, et al. "Replication of Cytomegalovirus in Human Arterial Smooth Muscle Cells." *J Virol* 56:3 (1985): 839–845. Morre, S.A., W. Stooker, W.K. Lagrand, et al. "Microorganisms in the Aetiology of Atherosclerosis." *J Clin Pathol* 53:9 (2000): 647–654.

37. Ooboshi, H., C.D. Rios, Y. Chu, et al. "Augmented Adenovirus-mediated Gene Transfer to Atherosclerotic Vessels." *Arterioscler Thromb Vasc Biol* 17:9 (1997): 1786–1792.

38. Ellis, R.W. "Infection and Coronary Heart Disease." *J Med Microbiol* 46:7 (1997): 535–539. Mattila, K.J., V.V. Valtonen, M.S. Nieminen, et al. "Role of Infection as a Risk Factor for Atherosclerosis, Myocardial Infarction, and Stroke." *Clin Infect Dis* 26:3 (1998): 719–734.

39. Chiu, B. "Multiple Infections in Carotid Atherosclerotic Plaques." *Am Heart J* 138:5 Part 2 (1999): S534–S536. Vercellotti, G.M. "Overview of Infections and Cardiovascular Diseases." *J Allergy Clin Immunol* 108:4 Suppl (2001): S117–S120.

40. Wanishsawad, C., Y.F. Zhou, S.E. Epstein. "*Chlamydia pneumoniae*-induced Transactivation of the Major Immediate Early Promoter of Cytomegalovirus: Potential Synergy of Infectious Agents in the Pathogenesis of Atherosclerosis." *J Infect Dis* 181:2 (2000): 787–790. Burnett, M.S., C.A. Gaydos, G.E. Madico, et al. "Atherosclerosis in ApoE Knockout Mice Infected with Multiple Pathogens." *J Infect Dis* 183:2 (2001): 226–231. Watt, S., B. Aesch, P. Lanotte, et al. "Viral and Bacterial DNA in Carotid Atherosclerotic Lesions." *Eur J Clin Microbiol Infect Dis* 22:2 (2003): 99–105. Virok, D., Z. Kis, L. Kari, et al. "*Chlamydophila pneumoniae* and Human Cytomegalovirus in Atherosclerotic Carotid Plaques—Combined Presence and Possible Interactions." *Acta Microbiol Immunol Hungary* 53:1 (2006): 35–50.

41. Espinola-Klein, C., H.J. Rupprecht, S. Blankenberg, et al. "Impact of Infectious Burden on Extent and Long-term Prognosis of Atherosclerosis." *Circulation* 105:1 (2002): 15–21. Espinola-Klein, C., H.J. Rupprecht, S. Blankenberg, et al. "Impact of Infectious Burden on Progression of Carotid Atherosclerosis." *Stroke* 33:11 (2002): 2581–2586. Auer, J., M. Leitinger, R. Berent, et al. "Influenza A and B IgG Seropositivity and Coronary Atherosclerosis Assessed by Angiography." *Heart Dis* 4:6 (2002): 349–354.

42. Speir, E. "Cytomegalovirus Gene Regulation by Reactive Oxygen Species. Agents in Atherosclerosis." *Ann NY Acad Sci* 899 (2000): 363–374.

43. Epstein, S.E., Y.F. Zhou, J. Zhu. "Infection and Atherosclerosis: Emerging Mechanistic Paradigms." *Circulation* 100:4 (1999): e20–e28.

44. Kariuki Njenga, M., and C.A. Dangler. "Endothelial MHC Class II Antigen Expression and Endarteritis Associated with Marek's Disease Virus Infection in Chickens." *Vet Pathol* 32:4 (1995): 403–411.

45. Fabricant, C.G., J. Fabricant, M.M. Litrenta, et al. "Virus-induced Atherosclerosis." *J Exp Med* 148:1 (1978): 335–340. Minick, C.R., C.G. Fabricant, J. Fabricant, et al. "Atheroarteriosclerosis Induced by Infection with a Herpesvirus." *Am J Pathol* 96:3 (1979): 673–706. Fabricant, C.G., J. Fabricant, C.R. Minick, et al. "Herpesvirus-induced Atherosclerosis in Chickens." *Fed Proc* 42:8 (1983): 2476–2479. Hajjar, D.P., D.J. Falcone, C.G. Fabricant, et al.

"Altered Cholesteryl Ester Cycle is Associated with Lipid Accumulation in Herpesvirus-infected Arterial Smooth Muscle Cells." *J Biol Chem* 260:10 (1985): 6124–6128.

46. Fabricant, C.G., and J. Fabricant. "Atherosclerosis Induced by Infection with Marek's Disease Herpesvirus in Chickens." *Am Heart J* 138:5 Part 2 (1999): S465–S468.

47. Shih, J.C., R. Pyrzak, J.S. Guy. "Discovery of Noninfectious Viral Genes Complementary to Marek's Disease Herpes Virus in Quail Susceptible to Cholesterol-induced Atherosclerosis." *J Nutr* 119:2 (1989): 294–298.

48. Span, A.H., G. Grauls, F. Bosman, et al. "Cytomegalovirus Infection Induces Vascular Injury in the Rat." *Atherosclerosis* 93:1-2 (1992): 41–52. Span, A.H., P.M. Frederik, G. Grauls, et al. "CMV-induced Vascular Injury: An Electron-microscopic Study in the Rat." *In Vivo* 7:6A (1993): 567–573.

49. Berencsi, K., V. Endresz, D. Klurfeld, et al. "Early Atherosclerotic Plaques in the Aorta following Cytomegalovirus Infection of Mice." *Cell Adhes Commun* 5:1 (1998): 39–47. Hsich, E., Y.F. Zhou, B. Paigen, et al. "Cytomegalovirus Infection Increases Development of Atherosclerosis in Apolipoprotein-E Knockout Mice." *Atherosclerosis* 156:1 (2001): 23–28.

50. Benditt, E.P., T. Barrett, J.K. McDougall. "Viruses in the Etiology of Atherosclerosis." *Proc Natl Acad Sci USA* 80:20 (1983): 6386–6389.

51. Melnick, J.L., E. Adam, M.E. Debakey. "Cytomegalovirus and Atherosclerosis." *Eur Heart J* 14:Suppl K (1993): 30–38. Hendrix, M.G., M.M. Salimans, C.P. van Boven, et al. "High Prevalence of Latently Present Cytomegalovirus in Arterial Walls of Patients Suffering from Grade III Atherosclerosis." *Am J Pathol* 136:1 (1990): 23–28. Hendrix, M.G., M. Daemen, C.A. Bruggeman. "Cytomegalovirus Nucleic Acid Distribution within the Human Vascular Tree." *Am J Pathol* 138:3 (1991): 563–567. Vercellotti, G.M. "Effects of Viral Activation of the Vessel Wall on Inflammation and Thrombosis." *Blood Coagul Fibrinolysis* 9:Suppl 2 (1998): S3–S6. Hu, W., J. Liu, S. Niu, et al. "Prevalence of CMV in Arterial Walls and Leukocytes in Patients with Atherosclerosis." *Chin Med J (England)* 114:11 (2001): 1208–1210.

52. Tanaka, S., Y. Toh, R. Mori, et al. "Possible Role of Cytomegalovirus in the Pathogenesis of Inflammatory Aortic Diseases: A Preliminary Report." *J Vasc Surg* 16:2 (1992): 274–279. Yonemitsu, Y., K. Komori, K. Sueishi, et al. "Possible Role of Cytomegalovirus Infection in the Pathogenesis of Human Vascular Diseases." *Nippon Rinsho* 56:1 (1998): 102–108.

53. Melnick, J.L., B.L. Petrie, G.R. Dreesman, et al. "Cytomegalovirus Antigen within Human Arterial Smooth Muscle Cells." *Lancet* 2:8351 (1983): 644–647. Shih, J.C., and D.W. Kelemen. "Possible Role of Viruses in Atherosclerosis."

Adv Exp Med Biol 369 (1995): 89–98. Nerheim, P.L., J.L. Meier, M.A. Vasef, et al. "Enhanced Cytomegalovirus Infection in Atherosclerotic Human Blood Vessels." *Am J Pathol* 164:2 (2004): 589–600.

54. Melnick, J.L., C. Hu, J. Burek, et al. "Cytomegalovirus DNA in Arterial Walls of Patients with Atherosclerosis." *J Med Virol* 42:2 (1994): 170–174.

55. Hendrix, M.G., P.H. Dormans, P. Kitslaar, et al. "The Presence of Cytomegalovirus Nucleic Acids in Arterial Walls of Atherosclerotic and Nonatherosclerotic Patients." *Am J Pathol* 134:5 (1989): 1151–1157.

56. Biocina, B., I. Husedzinovic, Z. Sutlic, et al. "Cytomegalovirus Disease as a Possible Etiologic Factor for Early Atherosclerosis." *Coll Antropol* 23:2 (1999): 673–681.

57. Pahl, E., F.J. Fricker, J. Armitage, et al. "Coronary Arteriosclerosis in Pediatric Heart Transplant Survivors: Limitation of Long-term Survival." *J Pediatr* 116:2 (1990): 177–183.

58. Yamashiroya, H.M., L. Ghosh, R. Yang, et al. "Herpesviridae in the Coronary Arteries and Aorta of Young Trauma Victims." *Am J Pathol* 130:1 (1988): 71–79.

59. Bruggeman, C.A. "Does Cytomegalovirus Play a Role in Atherosclerosis?" *Herpes* 7:2 (2000): 51–54. Melnick, J.L., E. Adam, M.E. DeBakey. "Cytomegalovirus and Atherosclerosis." *Bioessays* 17:10 (1995): 899–903.

60. Dhaunsi, G.S., J. Kaur, R.B. Turner. "Role of NADPH Oxidase in Cytomegalovirus-induced Proliferation of Human Coronary Artery Smooth Muscle Cells." *J Biomed Sci* 10:5 (2003): 505–509.

61. Cheng, J.W., and N.G. Rivera. "Infection and Atherosclerosis—Focus on Cytomegalovirus and *Chlamydia pneumoniae*." *Ann Pharmacother* 32:12 (1998): 1310–1316. High, K.P. "Atherosclerosis and Infection Due to *Chlamydia pneumoniae* or Cytomegalovirus: Weighing the Evidence." *Clin Infect Dis* 28:4 (1999): 746–749.

62. Famularo, G., V. Trinchieri, G. Santini, et al. "Infections, Atherosclerosis, and Coronary Heart Disease." *Ann Ital Med Int* 15:2 (2000): 144–155. Fong, I.W. "Emerging Relations between Infectious Diseases and Coronary Artery Disease and Atherosclerosis." *Can Med Assoc J* 163:1 (2000): 49–56. Mussa, F.F., H. Chai, X. Wang, et al. "*Chlamydia pneumoniae* and Vascular Disease: An Update." *J Vasc Surg* 43:6 (2006): 1301–1307.

63. Kuo, C.C., A.M. Gown, E.P. Benditt, et al. "Detection of *Chlamydia pneumoniae* in Aortic Lesions of Atherosclerosis by Immunocytochemical Stain." *Arterioscler Thromb* 13:10 (1993): 1501–1504. Kuo, C.C., J.T. Grayston, L.A. Campbell, et al. "*Chlamydia pneumoniae* (TWAR) in Coronary Arteries of

Young Adults (15–34 Years Old)." *Proc Natl Acad Sci USA* 92:15 (1995): 6911–6914. Davidson, M., C.C. Kuo, J.P. Middaugh, et al. "Confirmed Previous Infection with *Chlamydia pneumoniae* (TWAR) and Its Presence in Early Coronary Atherosclerosis." *Circulation* 98:7 (1998): 628–633.

64. Muhlestein, J.B., E.H. Hammond, J.F. Carlquist, et al. "Increased Incidence of *Chlamydia* Species within the Coronary Arteries of Patients with Symptomatic Atherosclerotic versus Other Forms of Cardiovascular Disease." *J Am Coll Cardiol* 27:7 (1996): 1555–1561. Campbell, L.A., et al. "Detection of *Chlamydia pneumoniae* in Atherectomy Tissue from Patients with Symptomatic Coronary Artery Disease." In Orfila, J., G. Byrne, M. Chernesky, et al. (eds.). *Chlamydial Infections.* Bologna, Italy: Societa Editrice Esculapio, 1994, pp. 212–215. Maass, M., J. Gieffers, E. Krause, et al. "Poor Correlation between Microimmunofluorescence Serology and Polymerase Chain Reaction for Detection of Vascular *Chlamydia pneumoniae* Infection in Coronary Artery Disease Patients." *Med Microbiol Immunol* 187 (1998): 103–106.

65. Espinola-Klein, C., H.J. Rupprecht, S. Blankenberg, et al. "Are Morphological or Functional Changes in the Carotid Artery Wall Associated with *Chlamydia pneumoniae, Helicobacter pylori,* Cytomegalovirus, or Herpes Simplex Virus Infection?" *Stroke* 31:9 (2000): 2127–2133.

66. Jahromi, B.S., M.D. Hill, K. Holmes, et al. "*Chlamydia pneumoniae* and Atherosclerosis following Carotid Endarterectomy." *Can J Neurol Sci* 30:4 (2003): 333–339.

67. Subramanian, A.K., T.C. Quinn, T.S. Kickler, et al. "Correlation of *Chlamydia pneumoniae* Infection and Severity of Accelerated Graft Arteriosclerosis after Cardiac Transplantation." *Transplantation* 73:5 (2002): 761–764.

68. Kuo, C.C., J.T. Grayston, L.A. Campbell, et al. "Chlamydia Pneumoniae (TWAR) in Coronary Arteries of Young Adults (15–35 Years Old)." *Proc Natl Acad Sci USA* 92 (1995): 6911–6914.

69. Ngeh, J., V. Anand, S. Gupta. "*Chlamydia pneumoniae* and Atherosclerosis—What We Know and What We Don't." *Clin Microbiol Infect* 8:1 (2002): 2–13.

70. Fong, I.W., B. Chiu, E. Viira, et al. "Rabbit Model for *Chlamydia pneumoniae* Infection." *J Clin Microbiol* 35 (1997): 48–52. Laitinen, K., A. Laurila, L. Pyhala, et al. "*Chlamydia pneumoniae* Infection Induces Inflammatory Changes in the Aorta of Rabbits." *Infect Immun* 65 (1997): 4832–4835. Moazed, T.C., L.A. Campbell, M.E. Rosenfeld, et al. "*Chlamydia pneumoniae* Infection Accelerates the Progression of Atherosclerosis in Apolipoprotein (Apo E)-Deficient Mice." *J Infect Dis* 180 (1999): 238–241. Muhlestein, J.B., J.L. Anderson, E.H. Hammond, et al. "Infection with *Chlamydia pneumoniae* Accelerates the Devel-

opment of Atherosclerosis and Treatment with Azithromycin Prevents It in a Rabbit Model." *Circulation* 97:7 (1998): 633–636.

71. Gurfinkel, E. "Link Between Intracellular Pathogens and Cardiovascular Diseases." *Clin Microbiol Infect* 4:Suppl 4 (1998): S33–S36.

72. Kalayoglu, M.V., B. Hoerneman, D. LaVerda, et al. "Cellular Oxidation of Low-Density Lipoprotein by *Chlamydia pneumoniae*." *J Infect Dis* 180 (1999): 780–790.

73. Shi, Y., and O. Tokunaga. "Herpesvirus (HSV-1, EBV and CMV) Infections in Atherosclerotic Compared with Non-atherosclerotic Aortic Tissue." *Pathol Intl* 52:1 (2002): 31–39.

74. Musiani, M., M.L. Zerbini, A. Muscari, et al. "Antibody Patterns against Cytomegalovirus and Epstein-Barr Virus in Human Atherosclerosis." *Microbiologica* 13:1 (1990): 35–41.

75. Tabib, A., C. Leroux, J.F. Mornex, et al. "Accelerated Coronary Atherosclerosis and Arteriosclerosis in Young Human-Immunodeficiency-Virus-Positive Patients." *Coron Artery Dis* 11:1 (2000): 41–46.

76. Rota, S. "*Mycobacterium tuberculosis* Complex in Atherosclerosis." *Acta Med Okayama* 59:6 (2005): 247–251.

77. Haraszthy, V.I., J.J. Zambon, M. Trevisan, et al. "Identification of Periodontal Pathogens in Atheromatous Plaques." *J Periodontol* 71:10 (2000): 1554–1560.

78. Fong, I.W. "Infections and Their Role in Atherosclerotic Vascular Disease." *J Am Dent Assoc* 133:Suppl (2002): 7S–13S.

79. Meurman, J.H., M. Sanz, S.J. Janket. "Oral Health, Atherosclerosis, and Cardiovascular Disease." *Crit Rev Oral Biol Med* 15:6 (2004): 403–413.

80. Suarna, C., R.T. Dean, J. May, et al. "Human Atherosclerotic Plaque Contains Both Oxidized Lipids and Relatively Large Amounts of Alpha-tocopherol and Ascorbate." *Arterioscler Thromb Vasc Biol* 15:10 (1995): 1616–1624.

81. Hickey, S., H.J. Roberts, and R.F. Cathcart. "Dynamic Flow." *J Orthomolecular Med* 20:4 (2005): 237–244.

82. O'Brien, K.D., C.E. Alpers, J.E. Hokanson, et al. "Oxidation-specific Epitopes in Human Coronary Atherosclerosis are Not Limited to Oxidized Low-density Lipoprotein." *Circulation* 94:6 (1996): 1216–1225. Westhuyzen, J. "The Oxidation Hypothesis of Atherosclerosis: An Update." *Ann Clin Lab Sci* 27:1 (1997): 1–10. Reaven, P.D., and J.L. Witztum. "Oxidized Low-density Lipoproteins in Atherogenesis: Role of Dietary Modification." *Annu Rev Nutr* 16 (1996): 51–71. Meagher, E., and D.J. Rader. "Antioxidant Therapy and Ath-

erosclerosis: Animal and Human Studies." *Trends Cardiovasc Med* 11:3–4 (2001): 162–165.

83. Cooke, J.P. "Is Atherosclerosis an Arginine Deficiency Disease?" *J Investig Med* 46 (1998): 377–380.

84. Tapiero, H., G. Mathe, P. Couvreur, et al. "Arginine." *Biomed Pharmacother* 56 (2002): 439–445. Preli, R.B., K.P. Klein, D.M. Herrington. "Vascular Effects of Dietary L-Arginine Supplementation." *Atherosclerosis* 162 (2002): 1–15. Tiefenbacher, C.P. "Tetrahydrobiopterin: A Critical Cofactor for eNOS and a Strategy in the Treatment of Endothelial Dysfunction?" *Am J Physiol Heart Circ Physiol* 280 (2001): H2484–H2488.

85. van Hinsbergh, V.W. "NO or H_2O_2 for Endothelium-dependent Vasorelaxation: Tetrahydrobiopterin Makes the Difference." *Arterioscler Thromb Vasc Biol* 21 (2001): 719–721.

86. Lehr, H.A., G. Germann, G.P. McGregor, et al. "Consensus Meeting on 'Relevance of Parenteral Vitamin C in Acute Endothelial-dependent Pathophysiological Conditions (EDPC)'." *Eur J Med Res* 11:12 (2006): 516–526.

87. Clementi, E., G.C. Brown, M. Feelisch. "Persistent Inhibition of Cell Respiration by Nitric Oxide: Crucial Role of S-Nitrosylation of Mitochondrial Complex 1 and Protective Action of Glutathione." *Proc Natl Acad Sci USA* 95 (1998): 7631–7636. Mogi, M., K. Kinpara, A. Kondo, et al. "Involvement of Nitric Oxide and Biopterin in Proinflammatory Cytokine-induced Apoptotic Cell Death in Mouse Osteoblastic Cell Line MC3T3." *Biochem Pharmacol* 58 (1999): 649–654. Bouton, C. "Nitrosative and Oxidative Modulation of Iron Regulatory Proteins." *Cell Mol Life Sci* 55 (1999): 1043–1053. Donnini, S., and M. Ziche. "Constitutive and Inducible Nitric Oxide Synthase: Role in Angiogenesis." *Antioxid Redox Signal* 4 (2002): 817–823.

88. Anderson, T.J. "Assessment and Treatment of Endothelial Dysfunction in Humans." *J Am Coll Cardiol* 34 (1999): 631–638. Watts, G.F., D.A. Playford, K.D. Croft, et al. "Coenzyme Q(10) Improves Endothelial Dysfunction of the Brachial Artery in Type II Diabetes Mellitus." *Diabetologia* 45 (2002): 420–426.

89. Cooke, J.P. "Does ADMA Cause Endothelial Dysfunction?" *Arterioscler Thromb Vasc Biol* 20 (2000): 2032–2037. Mukherjee, S., S.D. Coaxum, M. Maleque, et al. "Effects of Oxidized Low-density Lipoprotein on Nitric Oxide Synthetase and Protein Kinase C Activities in Bovine Endothelial Cells." *Cell Mol Biol* 47 (2001): 1051–1058.

90. Kirsch, M., H.G. Korth, R. Sustmann, et al. "The Pathobiochemistry of Nitrogen Dioxide." *Biol Chem* 383 (2002): 389–399. Chaudiere, J., and R. Ferrari-Iliou. "Intracellular Antioxidants: From Chemical to Biochemical Mechanisms." *Food Chem Toxicol* 37 (1999): 949–962. Regoli, F., and G.W. Winston.

"Quantification of Total Oxidant Scavenging Capacity of Antioxidants for Peroxynitrite, Peroxyl Radicals, and Hydroxyl Radicals." *Toxicol Appl Pharmacol* 156 (1999): 96–105.

91. Ceriello, A. "New Insights on Oxidative Stress and Diabetic Complications May Lead to a "Causal" Antioxidant Therapy." *Diabetes Care* 26 (2003): 1589–1596. Trujillo, M., and R. Radi. "Peroxynitrite Reaction with the Reduced and the Oxidized Forms of Lipoic Acid: New Insights into the Reaction of Peroxynitrite with Thiols." *Arch Biochem Biophys* 397 (2002): 91–98. Nakagawa, H., E. Sumiki, M. Takusagawa, et al. "Scavengers for Peroxynitrite: Inhibition of Tyrosine Nitration and Oxidation with Tryptamine Derivatives, Alpha-lipoic Acid and Synthetic Compounds." *Chem Pharm Bull* 48 (2000): 261–265. Whiteman, M., H. Tritschler, B. Halliwell. "Protection against Peroxynitrite-dependent Tyrosine Nitration and Alpha-1-antiproteinase Inactivation by Oxidized and Reduced Lipoic Acid." *FEBS Lett* 379 (1996): 74–76. Packer, L., K. Kraemer, G. Rimbach. "Molecular Aspects of Lipoic Acid in the Prevention of Diabetes Complications." *Nutrition* 17 (2001): 888–895.

92. Schopfer, F., N. Riobo, M.C. Carreras, et al. "Oxidation of Ubiquinol by Peroxynitrite: Implications for Protection of Mitochondria against Nitrosative Damage." *Biochem J* 349 (2003): 35–42.

93. Kjoller-Hansen, L., S. Boesgaard, J.B. Laursen, et al. "Importance of Thiols (SH Group) in the Cardiovascular System." *Ugeskr Laeger* 155 (1993): 3642–3645. Ferrari, R., C. Ceconi, S. Curello, et al. "Oxygen Free Radicals and Myocardial Damage: Protective Role of Thiol-containing Agents." *Am J Med* 91 (1991): 95S–105S. Cheung, P.Y., W. Wang, R. Schulz. "Glutathione Protects against Myocardial Ischemia-reperfusion Injury by Detoxifying Peroxynitrite." *J Mol Cell Cardiol* 32 (2000): 1669–1678. Deneke, S.M. "Thiol-based Antioxidants." *Curr Top Cell Regul* 36 (2000): 151–180. Del Corso, A., P.G. Vilardo, M. Cappiello, et al. "Physiological Thiols as Promoters of Glutathione Oxidation and Modifying Agents in Protein S Thiolation." *Arch Biochem Biophys* 397 (2002): 392–398. Ramires, P.R., and L.L. Ji. "Glutathione Supplementation and Training Increases Myocardial Resistance to Ischemia-reperfusion in Vivo." *Am J Physiol Heart Circ Physiol* 281 (2001): H679–H688.

94. Chaudiere, J., and R. Ferrari-Iliou. "Intracellular Antioxidants: From Chemical to Biochemical Mechanisms." *Food Chem Toxicol* 37 (1999): 949–962.

95. McCarty, M.F. "Oxidants Downstream from Superoxide Inhibit Nitric Oxide Production by Vascular Endothelium—A Key Role for Selenium-dependent Enzymes in Vascular Health." *Med Hypotheses* 53 (1999): 315–325.

96. Terao, J., S. Yamaguchi, M. Shirai, et al. "Protection by Quercetin and Quercetin 3-O-beta-D-glucuronide of Peroxynitrite-induced Antioxidant Consumption in Human Plasma Low-density Lipoprotein." *Free Radical Res* 35

(2001): 925–931. Haenen, G.R., J.B. Paquay, R.E. Korthouwer, et al. "Peroxynitrite Scavenging by Flavonoids." *Biochem Biophys Res Commun* 236 (1997): 591–593.

97. Hickey, S., H.J. Roberts, R.F. Cathcart. "Dynamic Flow." *J Orthomolecular Med* 20:4 (2005): 237–244.

98. Simon, E., J. Gariepy, A. Cogny, et al. "Erythrocyte, but Not Plasma, Vitamin E Concentration is Associated with Carotid Intima-media Thickening in Asymptomatic Men at Risk for Cardiovascular Disease." *Atherosclerosis* 159 (2001): 193–200. Andreeva-Gateva, P. "Antioxidant Vitamins—Significance for Preventing Cardiovascular Diseases. Part 1. Oxidized Low-density Lipoproteins and Atherosclerosis; Antioxidant Dietary Supplementation—Vitamin E." *Vutr Boles* 32 (2000): 11–18. Bolton-Smith, C., M. Woodward, H. Tunstall-Pedoe. "The Scottish Heart Health Study. Dietary Intake by Food Frequency Questionnaire and Odds Ratios for Coronary Heart Disease Risk. II. The Antioxidant Vitamins and Fibre." *Eur J Clin Nutr* 46 (1992): 85–93. Eichholzer, M., H.B. Stahelin, K.F. Gey. "Inverse Correlation between Essential Antioxidants in Plasma and Subsequent Risk to Develop Cancer, Ischemic Heart Disease and Stroke, Respectively: 12-Year Follow-up of the Prospective Basel Study." *EXS* 62 (1992): 398–410. O'Byrne, D., S. Grundy, L. Packer, et al. "Studies of LDL Oxidation Following Alpha-, Gamma-, or Delta-tocotrienyl Acetate Supplementation of Hypercholesterolemic Humans." *Free Radical Biol Med* 29 (2000): 834–845.

99. Knekt, P., R. Jarvinen, A. Reunanen, et al. "Flavonoid Intake and Coronary Mortality in Finland: A Cohort Study." *Br Med J* 312 (1996): 478–481. Formica, J.V., and W. Regelson. "Review of the Biology of Quercetin and Related Bioflavonoids." *Food Chem Toxicol* 33 (1995): 1061–1080. Kolchin, I.N., N.P. Maksiutina, P.P. Balanda, et al. "The Cardioprotective Action of Quercetin in Experimental Occlusion and Reperfusion of the Coronary Artery in Dogs." *Farmakol Toksikol* 54 (1991): 20–23.

100. Zhang, W.J., and B. Frei. "Alpha-lipoic Acid Inhibits TNF-Alpha-induced NF-KappaB Activation and Adhesion Molecule Expression in Human Aortic Endothelial Cells." *FASEB J* 15 (2001): 2423–2432. Kunt, T., T. Forst, A. Wilhelm, et al. "Alpha-lipoic Acid Reduces Expression of Vascular Cell Adhesion Molecule-1 and Endothelial Adhesion of Human Monocytes after Stimulation with Advanced Glycation End Products." *Clin Sci* 96 (1999): 75–82. Bierhaus, A., S. Chevion, M. Chevion, et al. "Advanced Glycation End Product–induced Activation of NF-KappaB is Suppressed by Alpha-lipoic Acid in Cultured Endothelial Cells." *Diabetes* 46 (1997): 1481–1490.

101. Hickey, S., and H. Roberts. *Ascorbate: The Science of Vitamin C.* Lulu Press, 2004.

Index

Blood glucose. *See* Blood sugar.
Blood plasma, 46
Blood pressure, high, 127–128,
    130–131, 139
Blood sugar, 46–47
Bowel tolerance, 51, 52, 62, 99,
    104, 107
Brighthope, Ian, 105
Bronchitis, 137

C
Calcium, 52, 58
Calcium oxalate stones, 58
Calories, 120
Cameron, Ewan, 33, 116
Cancer, x, xiii, 15, 33–34, 36, 71,
    85, 109–122, 144, 146. *See
    also* Tumors.
    basics of, 109–113
    breast, 113
    case study, 120–122
    lung, 64–66, 73, 113, 120–122
    prostate, 113
Cancer and Vitamin C, 33
Carbohydrates, low intake, 120
Carcinogenesis, 116–117
Carcinomas, 113–114
Cardiovascular disease, 34, 73,
    123–142
"Cargo Cult" science, 74–75
Carnitine, 2
Cataracts, 17–18
Cathcart, Robert F., III, x, 6, 9,
    28, 41, 49, 52, 60–61, 79,
    82, 86, 98, 99, 101, 104,
    105, 106, 107, 108, 139,
    142, 143
Cells, 109–113

smooth muscle, 132–133, 136,
    140
suicide, 111–113
Chemotherapy, 119–120
Children, 28–30
Children's Doctor, The, 29
Chlamydia pneumoniae, 134,
    136–138
Chlamydia trachomatis, 136
Cholera, 69–70
Cholesterol, 2, 129, 130, 140,
    141
    low-density (LDL), 128, 134
Chromosomes, 9–10
Circulation system, 123–124
Citrulline, 141
Cochrane Collaboration, 77, 79,
    80–82
Coenyzme Q$_{10}$, 98, 139, 140, 141
Coherence, 66
Colds, ix, 36, 75, 77–78, 85, 99,
    145
Collagen, x, 2, 13, 32–33
Columbia University College of
    Physicians and Surgeons, 31
Consistency, 66
Contraceptives, 80
Conventional medicine vs.
    Vitamin C, 63–90
Coxsackie B4 virus, 134
C-reactive protein. *See* CRP.
Crick, Frances, 72
CRP, 128
Cytomegalovirus, 134, 136, 137,
    138

D
Darwin, Charles, 32, 67, 88

About the Authors

Steve Hickey has a B.A. (math and science) from the Open University, membership of the Institute of Biology by examination in pharmacology, and is a chartered biologist and a former member of the British Computer Society. He did research into ultra-high-resolution computerized tomography (CT) body scanning, leading the physics team in Europe's first clinical magnetic resonance (MR) imaging unit at Manchester Medical School. He has over 100 scientific publications, covering a variety of disciplines. Currently, he is a member of the biology department of Staffordshire University.

Andrew W. Saul has over 30 years of experience in natural health education. He taught nutrition, health science, and cell biology at the college level for nine years. He is chairman of the Independent Vitamin Safety Review Panel, editor of the *Orthomolecular Medicine News Service,* and assistant editor of the *Journal of Orthomolecular Medicine.* He is the author of *Doctor Yourself* and *Fire Your Doctor!* (both available from Basic Health Publications). His popular peer-reviewed, non-commercial natural healing website is www.DoctorYourself.com.

CPSIA information can be obtained
at www.ICGtesting.com
Printed in the USA
LVOW10*2324210517
535374LV00021B/729/P